Fettouma Mazari
Alfendi Sakr

Infectious and post-traumatic emergencies in ophthalmology

Fettouma Mazari
Alfendi Sakr

Infectious and post-traumatic emergencies in ophthalmology

ScienciaScripts

Publisher:
Sciencia Scripts
is a trademark of
Dodo Books Indian Ocean Ltd. and OmniScriptum S.R.L publishing group

120 High Road, East Finchley, London, N2 9ED, United Kingdom
Str. Armeneasca 28/1, office 1, Chisinau MD-2012, Republic of Moldova, Europe
Printed at: see last page
ISBN: 978-620-7-40376-9

SUMMARY

Emergency ophthalmological conditions account for the highest percentage of ophthalmology consultations. Ophthalmological emergencies constitute a varied group of pathologies that any specialist or general practitioner may encounter in their daily practice. A good diagnostic approach based on a thorough history, the results of a clinical examination and the results of the investigations carried out will determine the quality of the treatment. The ocular symptoms that motivate patients to seek emergency care vary greatly, and are closely related to the pathology in question. It may be a case of ocular trauma, the symptoms of which will obviously be more varied, associating a drop in visual acuity, a red eye, lacrimation or even more. It may also be a case of a drop in visual acuity, lacrimation, a red eye, photophobia or diplopia. The aim of this book is to provide an overview of the main emergencies encountered in ophthalmology.

TABLE OF CONTENTS

INTRODUCTION

An urgent medical or surgical condition is defined as one that needs to be treated without delay (1). There are a wide variety of emergency conditions in ophthalmology, and all doctors must be able to recognise them so that they can be treated in good time. The general practitioner is most often the first to see the patient, and is the first point of call for care. His role is well known, and is based essentially on the collection of functional signs, the results of the interview and the signs of the ophthalmological examination that he has carried out with the very limited resources at his disposal, enabling him to make appropriate referrals for treatment (2).

The prevalence of ophthalmological emergencies compared with general emergencies around the world varies from 1 to 5% in France (3), from 1.46 to 6.1% in the United Kingdom (4) and from 1.5 to 2.6% in the United States (5). Ophthalmological emergencies had a prevalence of 4.3% according to Odoulami et al (6). A distinction is generally made between traumatic and non-traumatic ophthalmological emergencies.

The ocular symptoms that motivate patients to seek emergency care vary greatly, and are closely related to the pathology in question. It may be a case of ocular trauma, the symptoms of which will obviously be more varied, associating a drop in visual acuity, a red eye, lacrimation or even more. It may also be a case of a drop in visual acuity, lacrimation, a red eye, photophobia or diplopia.
In this work, we present our experience of ophthalmological emergencies encountered in our daily practice. These emergencies are post-traumatic, infectious and vascular in origin.

<h1 align="center">EYE INJURIES</h1>

1- Introduction :

The role of trauma in the statistics on the causes of blindness in the world is often underestimated compared with other causes such as cataracts, diabetic retinopathy, glaucoma, etc. The WHO (World Health Organisation) lists some 55 million cases of ocular trauma per year, responsible for 19 million cases of monocular blindness worldwide, 32 to 75% of which occur in children (1) (2).

Ocular trauma often has serious socio-professional, medico-legal and economic consequences, particularly as it affects young people, usually men, in the midst of their careers (5).

Tissue damage is closely related to the circumstances of the trauma and the type of trauma, which may be a contusion, an open trauma with or without an intraocular foreign body, or a physical or chemical burn.

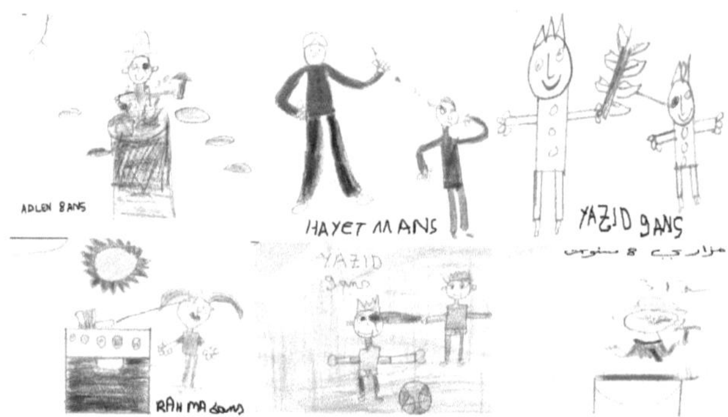

Figure 1: Children's imaginations of different situations that can lead to eye trauma (Iconography by Pr Mazari).

2- Pathophysiology of ocular trauma in general:

The eyeball is protected by the eyelids and the blink reflex, the bony orbit and the head's evasive reflex movements. Sometimes these defence systems are insufficient, in which case the eye may be exposed to trauma of some kind.

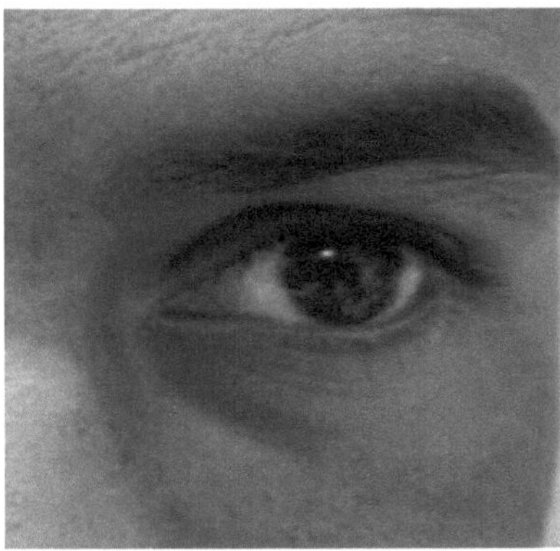

Figure 2: External configuration of the eyeball and its appendages
(Iconography by Pr Mazari).

In the event of contusion, the eye is subjected to a shock wave from front to back that can damage all ocular and surrounding structures (cornea, crystalline lens, anterior chamber and retina). The causal agent is most often foam.In the case of perforating trauma, the causal agent is a sharp object, and tissue damage will depend on the portal of entry and the speed of penetration of the object (5).

3- Questioning :

The interview will enable us to :
*Determine the circumstances of the accident: The most common accidents are accidents at work, accidents in the home and sporting accidents (5), followed by assault-related injuries. Accidents on the public highway have become rarer since the introduction of compulsory wearing of safety belts.

This said, the airbag is sometimes blamed for eye contusions.
*Determine the nature of the traumatic agent (appearance, composition and temperature). The traumatic agent is an essential element in determining the functional prognosis.
* Specify the patient's ophthalmological and general pathological history, especially if a general anaesthetic is envisaged (age, tetanus vaccination status, time of last meal, any allergies, etc.).

4- Clinical examination :

The initial examination can be carried out by a general practitioner, especially in regions where there is no ophthalmologist available. However, certain clinical signs require the patient to be referred to a specialist: a drop in visual acuity, major palpebral oedema preventing examination of the eyeball, chemosis, hypotonia, pupillary deformation or hyphaema.

The clinical examination should follow these steps:
▶ Distance and near visual acuity must be assessed (forensic value).
▶ The examination should focus on external structures such as the eyelids

orbital framework, adnexa and conjunctival cul-de-sacs.
▶ Biomicroscopic examination is essential, enabling us to correctly
examine the various structures of the eyeball: the conjunctiva, the
cornea, then the anterior chamber, the iris and the lens.
▶ Intraocular pressure is most often measured by palpebral touch, when it is not possible to measure tone using the GOLDMAN aplanation, as in the case of major palpebral oedema associated with intense pain or corneal disorder. Hypotonia points to perforating trauma and hypertonia to anterior chamber haemorrhage or hyphaema).
▶ When possible, a fundus examination can reveal

depending on the type of trauma (vitreous haemorrhage, the presence of a intraocular foreign body, a retinal lesion (Berlin oedema, retinal haemorrhages, tears, retinal dialysis after a contusion or retinal wound after a perforating trauma)...
▶ A descriptive certificate is often drawn up at the end of the initial examination, which is binding on the practitioner first and foremost, and useful to the patient in asserting his or her social, employment, civil or criminal rights.

Birmingham's international classification separates trauma that respects the integrity of the eyeball from trauma that breaks through its full thickness wall (cornea or sclera) [3,9] .

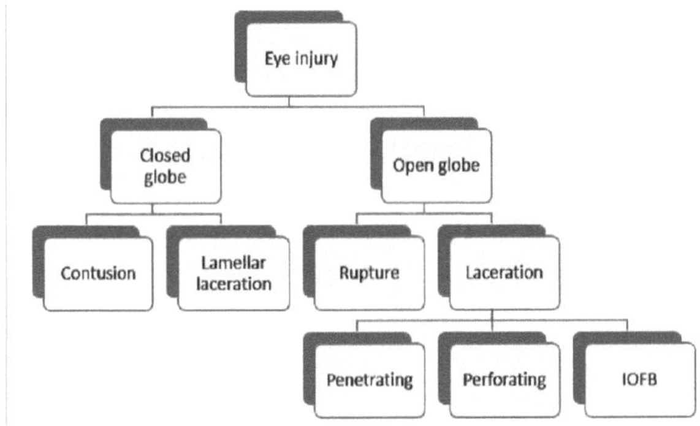

Figure 3: The Birmingham International Classification of Ocular Trauma

5- Additional tests :

Further tests will be ordered depending on the clinical context (contusive trauma or perforating trauma with or without an intraocular foreign body).

▶ Standard X-rays :

In theory, they are compulsory (for medico-legal reasons) in the event of a suspected eye injury, in order to detect the presence of a radio-opaque foreign body and locate it. The following 3 X-rays should be requested

•Blondeau: clear the 2 orbits of the bone,

•X-ray of the orbit in profile (diseased side against the plate, to limit magnifications),

•X-ray focusing on the orbits in the 4 directions of view (up, down, right and left).

▶ B-mode ocular ultrasound :

It will be requested every time there is a loss of transparency of the media, but only in contusive trauma. On the other hand, in perforating trauma, it is most often deferred due to the risk of infection and aggravation of the trauma, as it requires a probe to be placed in the eyeball.

▶ CT scan or CT densitometry:

It is the examination of choice in ocular trauma, second only to plain x-rays. It will confirm or rule out the existence of an associated bone fracture or an intraocular foreign body. It should be remembered that MRI is formally contraindicated in cases where a metallic foreign body is suspected.

A- Blunt trauma :

All ocular structures may be involved, and they are most often multiple and simultaneous, or appear at a distance from the date of the trauma.

Trauma to a closed globe is more frequent: 40 to 92% of cases, depending on the study [3]. The prognosis is better than for trauma to an open globe, as the globe is protected by the orbital frame, but the trauma is sometimes more serious, causing lesions in the anterior segment (hyphema, disinsertion of the base of the iris, zonular rupture, lens dislocation or opacification, etc.) and the posterior segment (Berlin oedema, vitreoretinal lesions or even retinal detachment, which should be sought in predisposed patients such as myopes).) and the posterior segment (Berlin oedema, vitreoretinal lesions or even retinal detachment, which should be sought in predisposed patients such as myopes)(8).

■ The causal agent: this could be a ball, a stone thrown or, as is most often the case, a blow from a hand, as is the case in assaults.

■ Pathophysiology: Direct trauma to the surface of the eye will create a vectorial force directed towards the back of the orbital cavity and cause equatorial expansion of the eye, resulting in stretching. of the endocular structures, there will then be a backlash force directed in the opposite direction, causing compression of the vitreous and projecting the lens and iris forward, as well as the retina and choroid.

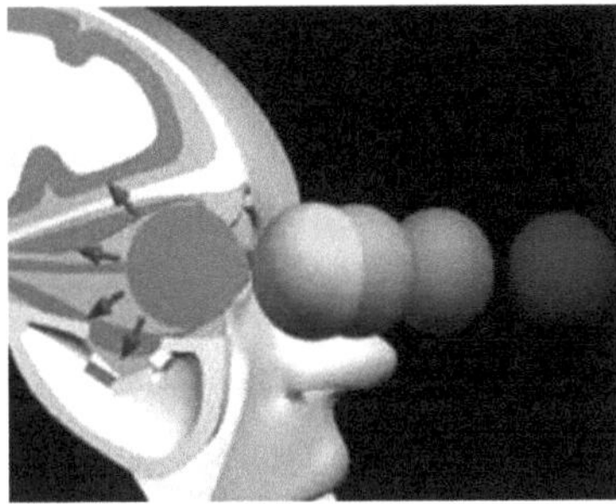

Figure 4: Contusive trauma caused by a tennis ball (literature collection)

Contusive trauma may involve the orbital region and its appendages or the eyeball.

1- CONTUSIVE TRAUMA TO THE ORBIT

Trauma to the orbit is very common in facial trauma, and this is of course closely related to its anatomical situation. These injuries mainly affect young people (7)(8), most of whom are men. The mechanisms of onset are variable, and the severity of the lesions is variable.depends on the intensity of the trauma and the traumatic agent involved. These include zygomatic and orbital floor fractures, fractures of the naso-ethmoid-maxillofronto-orbital complex (NEMFC) and craniofacial disjunctions of the Le Fort II and III types. These orbital traumas are often associated with lesions of the orbital contents (globe, oculomotor muscles and nerves, optic nerve) as well as the eyelids and lacrimal apparatus (9). The clinical examination will assess visual acuity, the statics of the eyeballs, looking for enophthalmos or exophthalmos, a decrease in ocular tone, oculomotricity, and the condition of the palpebral apparatus and lacrimal ducts. Computed tomography of the facial mass in millimetre slices allowing reconstruction in the three planes of space provides an exhaustive assessment of the lesions.

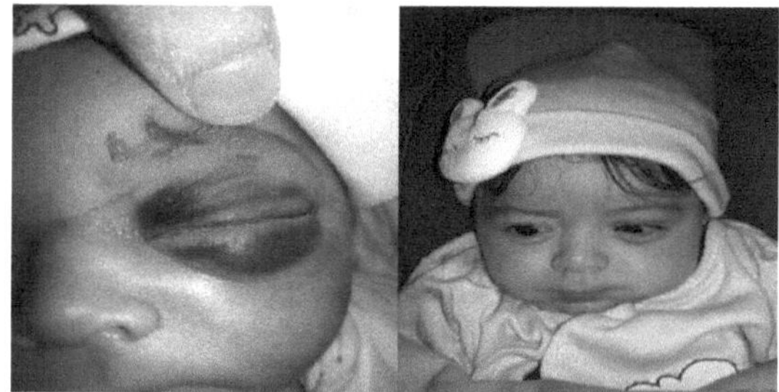

a b

Figure 5: a : Orbital haematoma in a newborn following an ill-adapted forceps during vaginal delivery. b: 3 months later, regression of lesions with no sequelae (Iconography by Pr Mazari).

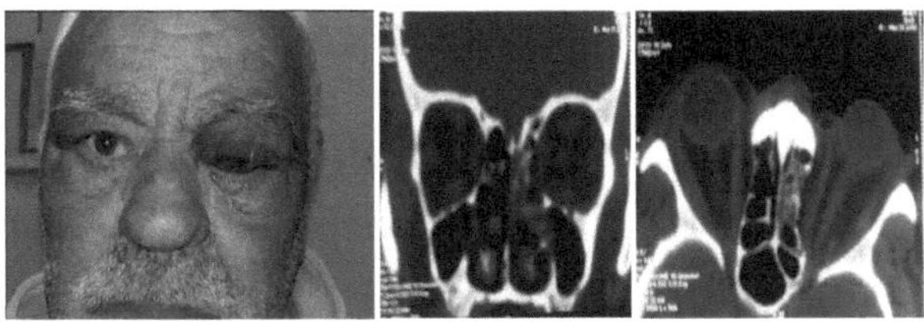

Figure 6: Fracture depression of the internal wall of the orbit with hematic filling of the homolateral ethmoidal cells and s/cutaneous emphysema MOM integrity. (Iconography by Pr Mazari).

Treatment remains urgent in cases of facial damage, with the aim of preserving visual function or even vital prognosis. In non-urgent situations, repair of fractures of the orbit is carried out remotely, to allow the oedema to subside. After reduction, osteosynthesis of orbital fractures is performed using screw plates. The walls of the orbit are repaired using plates made of resorbable materials, titanium grids or bone grafts.

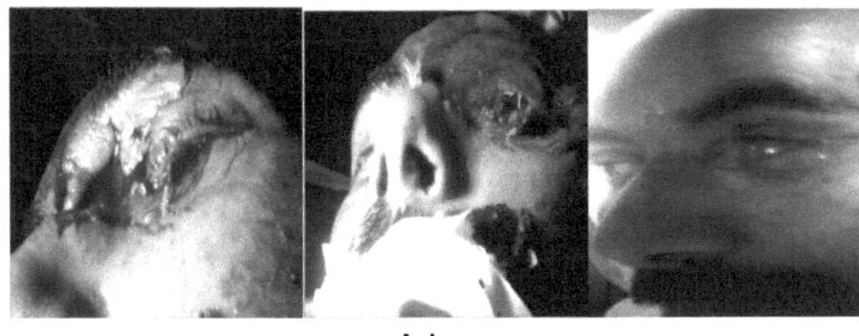

A b c

Figure 7 : Patient aged 37, victim of an accident at work (bursting of a chainsaw) resulting in orbito-palpebral dislocation and a shredded eyeball. Operated on for 4 hours with the aim of restoring anatomy.
A and b: Before surgery, c: the same patient 4 months later, satisfactory anatomical reconstruction (Iconography by Pr Mazari).

2- CONTUSIVE PALPEBRAL TRAUMA

Damage to the eyelids can occur in all cases of contusive or perforating ocular trauma. Their severity can range from a simple abrasion, haematoma or ecchymosis to major damage.

Questioning :
It will specify the mechanism of the trauma: contusion, frank section, tearing, dog bite or maxillofacial trauma. In all cases of palpebral trauma, the following should be considered:
- Abalancebetween lesion priorities inpolytrauma patients, especially head trauma patients.
- Look for a wound or contusion of the underlying globe,
- Look for a fracture of the underlying orbit.
- Assess the function of the levator eyelid muscle before putting the patient to sleep if suturing the wound requires a general anaesthetic.
- The examination must be very gentle, with no pressure applied in case there is a wound.
of the eyeball.

Types of palpebral wounds and their suture:

We can find :
- Parallel wounds at a distance from the free edge, which heal easily (lines

physiological) after a simple edge-to-edge suture.
- Wounds affecting the free edge need to be carefully sutured to prevent deformation and/or malposition of the eyelashes.
- Wound at the inner angle of the eyelids, always think of a section or tearing of the lacrimal canaliculi to be repaired by microsurgery.
- The upper eyelid wound may be associated with a section of the levator eyelid muscle, which must be carefully sutured by qualified personnel to avoid secondary ptosis.

- Check that you have been vaccinatedagainst tetanus and,if you have been bitten, contact the anti-rabies centre.

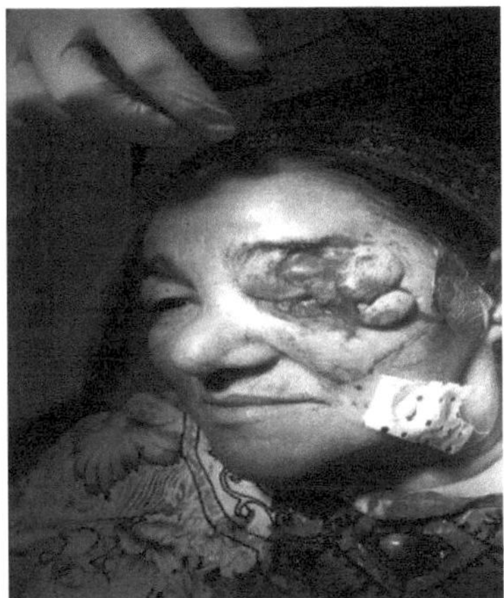

Figure 8: Palpebral damage in a woman after exposure to a bottle of deodorant (Iconography by Pr Mazari).

3- ANTERIOR SEGMENT CONTUSIONS

1- Conjunctival lesions :

Most often it is a haemorrhage, which may be minimal in the form of a red patch localised to part of the conjunctiva, or a true conjunctival haematoma involving the entire conjunctiva. If there is significant haemorrhage, a search must be made for an underlying wound or foreign body, depending on the circumstances of the trauma and the causal agent.

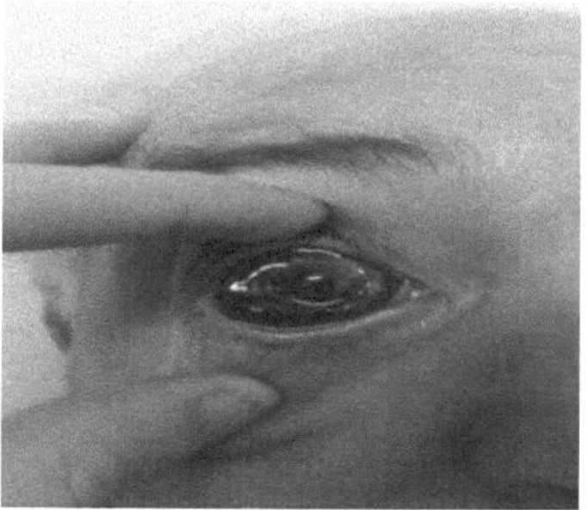

Figure 9: Conjunctival haematoma post-contusive to an elbow blow in a patient on anticoagulants (Iconography by Pr F Mazari).

▶ Treatment of conjunctival haemorrhage :
There is no specific treatment for conjunctival haemorrhage, which resolves spontaneously within 1 to 2 weeks depending on the extent of the haemorrhage. However, patients may be given NSAID-based eye drops such as indocollyre* and wetting agents.

2- Contusion of the cornea :

This erosion is revealed by instilling a drop of fluorescein, which colours the corneal lesion yellow-green. It can also be a severe contusion that can cause corneal edema with reduced visual acuity. The main symptom is pain, especially in adults, with the sensation of a foreign body, sometimes very severe, accompanied by photophobia and lacrimation. Examination shows conjunctival hyperhaemia, blepharospasm and lacrimation, associated with a drop in acuity if the erosion is central. For treatment, corneal erosion is treated with wetting agents and antiseptics in eye drops in order to avoid superinfection, with an ocular dressing until the erosion has healed. On the other hand, in the case of post-contusive corneal oedema, steroidal anti-inflammatory eye drops and ointments are used, always with wetting agents, for 10 to 15 days, with regular monitoring.

3- Contusion of the anterior chamber :

Hyphaemia, defined by the presence of a haematic level in the anterior chamber, is common and occurs immediately after trauma. It usually evolves spontaneously towards resorption, but there is a risk of recurrence of haemorrhage. Massive recurrent hyphaema may be responsible for ocular hypertonia, and if the hyphaema persists for more than a few days, it may be the cause of a haematic infiltration of the cornea, known as haematocornea, which is a brownish discolouration of the cornea by iron contained in the blood. It is usually irreversible.

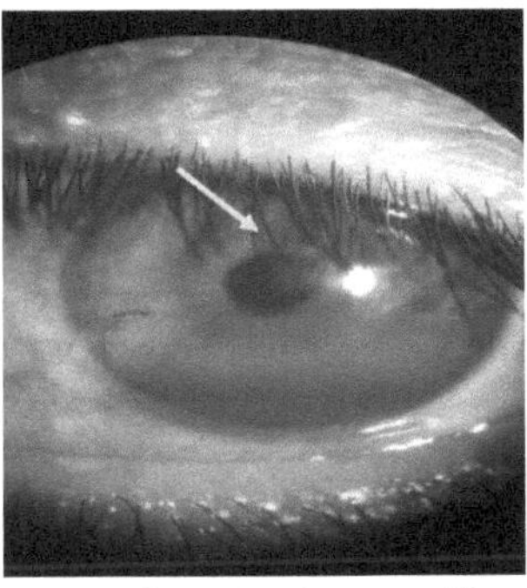

Figure 10: Hyphaema stage I contusive position (Iconography by Pr F Mazari).

The patient presents to emergency with a drop in visual acuity of varying intensity, depending on the level of haemorrhage in the anterior chamber. And if the hyphaema is associated with ocular hypertonia, the patient will also present with pain, which is usually very severe. For the treatment of hyphema, hospitalisation is the rule, in order to put the patient at strict rest. The patient should be given a course of fluids, with copious drinks to enable the blood in the anterior chamber to be washed out by rapid renewal of the aqueous humour. Treatment with NSAID- or corticosteroid-based eye drops can help reduce inflammation.

In the event of complications due to ocular hypertonia, a hypnotic treatment such as mannitol, which acts by dehydrating the vitreous, should be added.It is essential to monitor the patient daily by examining the anterior segment and measuring eye tone.If the hyphaema does not resolve after 7 to 10 days, with the possibility of ocular hypertonia appearing, the blood must be surgically evacuated in order to avoid haematocornea.

4- Contusion of the iris :

This may be iridodialysis, defined as a disinsertion of the iris at its base. Or a rupture of the sphincter of the iris or the edge of the pupil,

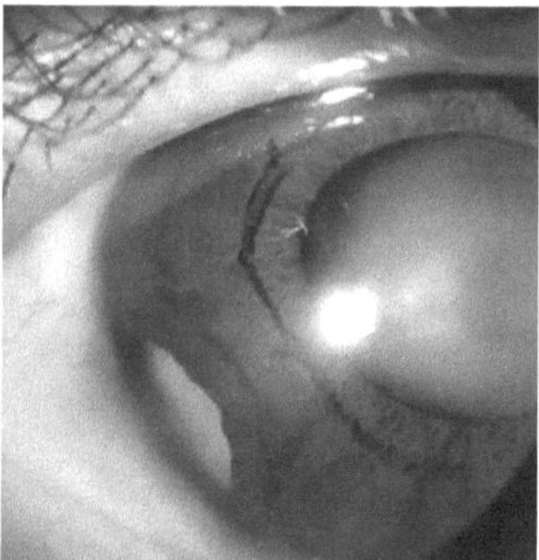

Figure11: Post-contusive dialysis using a ping-pong ball (Iconography by Pr Mazari).

There is no specific treatment for sphincter rupture. However, in the case of significant irido-dialysis, where the patient may have monocular diplopia, surgical treatment consists of reinserting the root of the iris at the point of disinsertion using a simple suture.

5- Contusion of the lens :

Damage to the crystalline lens is uncommon in contusions of the eyeball where the trauma is not very severe. On the other hand, in trauma with a strong impact, damage to the lens is almost constant, given the fragility of the zonular fibres. There will be either sub-luxation of the lens or dislocation of the lens either in the anterior chamber or in the vitreous. Contusive cataract: the onset of which is most often delayed by months or even years after the trauma.

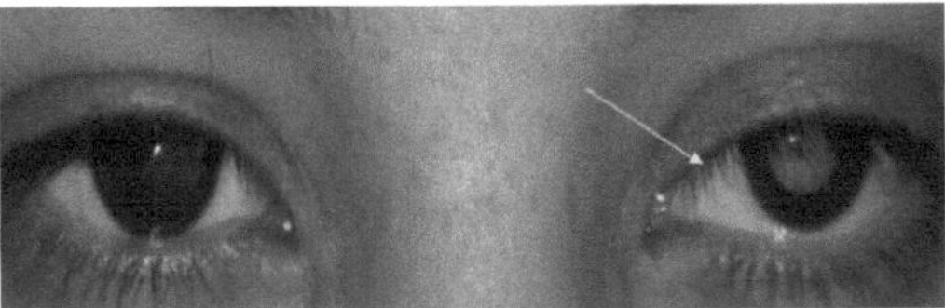

Figure 12: Post-traumatic white cataract in a child (Iconography by Pr Mazari).

Decreased visual acuity is the main reason for consultation in cases of lens damage. In the case of posterior dislocation of the lens, the drop in visual acuity will be very significant and occurs immediately after the trauma. However, in the case of dislocation of the crystalline lens in the anterior chamber, the picture is much more severe, as pupillary blocking occurs, causing major hypertonia and considerable pain. In the case of cataracts, the reduction in visual acuity is progressive and may last for years after the trauma. Lens lesions are treated surgically. In the case of subluxation of the lens, if it is minimal and vision is not impaired, simple monitoring can be carried out. However, in the case of complete dislocation, i.e. where the zonular fibres have been cut in their entirety, the lens will be extracted intra-capsularly and a scleral-fixed implant will be placed. In the case of a cataract, a phacoemulsification will be carried out with the insertion of a cataract. an implant in the posterior chamber.

4- CONTUSIONS OF THE POSTERIOR SEGMENT

Post-traumatic lesions of the posterior segment are more serious than those of the anterior segment because retinal damage compromises visual function to a greater extent. This may involve :

1- Post contusuf retinal oedema :

Retinal oedema of the posterior pole, also known as Berlin oedema, is responsible for an initial drop in visual acuity. It usually resolves, but can sometimes lead to the formation of a macular hole, with a severe and permanent reduction in visual acuity. Treatment is medical, using local and systemic corticosteroids, although their efficacy has not been proven.

2- Intravitreal haemorrhage due to vascular rupture traumatic retinal:

It is manifested by a drop in visual acuity of varying intensity depending on the concentration of haemorrhage in the vitreous gel. It generally progresses favourably, towards spontaneous resorption; when it prevents the retina from being seen, a B ultrasound should be performed to look for an associated retinal detachment. It generally progresses favourably, towards spontaneous resorption after 2 to 3 months; if this is not the case, surgical treatment by vitrectomy should be carried out.

3- Peripheral retinal tears :

In the event of any contusion of the eyeball, a three-mirror examination should be carried out, enabling the peripheral retina to be examined for retinal tears. In most cases, retinal disinsertion is found. These retinal tears can lead to retinal detachment, which can occur at a distance from the trauma, especially in at-risk subjects such as myopes.

Treatment: The treatment of these tears consists of performing a laser block as early as possible before the retinal detachment sets in, which is treated surgically.

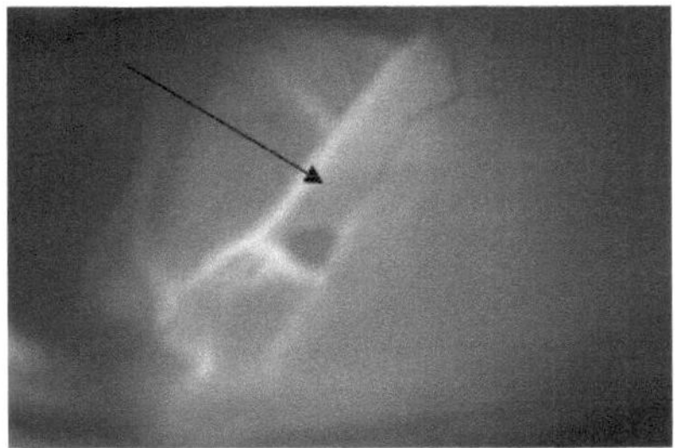

Figure 13; Retinal tear complicated by retinal detachment (Iconography by Pr Mazari).

4- Post contusive retinal detachment :

Post-contusive retinal detachment may be considered to have a better prognosis than retinal detachment caused by perforating trauma. Tears are most often peripheral, in the form of retinal disinsertions, which is why it is necessary to examine the retinal periphery with a three-mirror lens in search of a tear or disinsertion with a view to treating it with a laser in order to prevent retinal detachment.

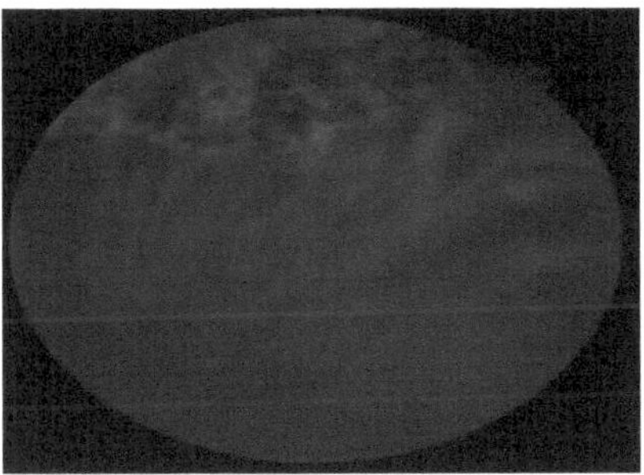

Figure 14: Laser treatment of a very peripheral retinal detachment (Iconography by Pr Mazari).

The treatment of retinal detachment by disinsertion involves an external indentation. It may also be a case of retinal detachment due to a post-contusive macular hole, in which case the prognosis is less favourable. Treatment involves vitrectomy.

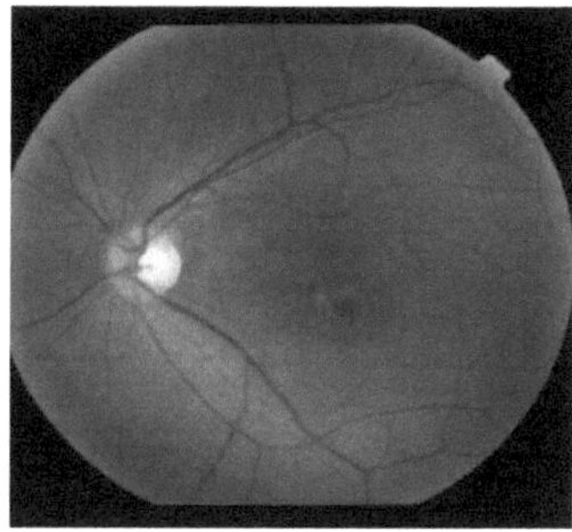

Figure 15:Retinography of a peripheral post-contusive macular hole
(Iconography by Pr Mazari)

B- Penetrating ocular trauma :

They are much more serious than blunt ocular trauma (10)(11). Lesions can range from a simple small corneal wound to the bursting of the eyeball. They are secondary to trauma by sharp objects. Imaging (X-rays, ultrasound, UBM, OCT, MRI) is essential, if not mandatory, for any open ocular trauma with a suspected intraocular foreign body (medicolegal interest).The damage may be mixed, combining wounds and contusions. There may be significant damage in the context of trauma to the face (work accidents, road accidents, disasters and acts of war), in which case the visual prognosis is only one element of the overall functional prognosis. Any trauma to the eye involves the visual prognosis.

1- Ocular wounds without intraocular foreign bodies :
1-1- Corneal wounds :

The shape and size of the wound will depend on the sharp object; it may be punctiform, as in the case of trauma by a thorn with effusion of the aqueous humour (positive Seidel), or very large, extending from one end of the cornea to the other, as in the case of trauma by a chisel or knife.

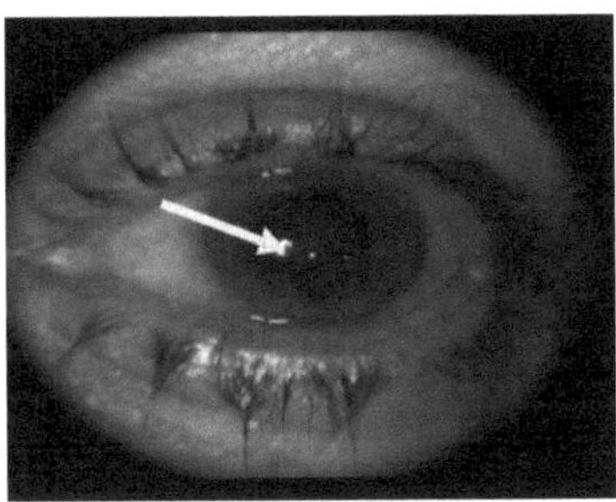

Figure 16: Corneal wound in a child, caused by the cap of a pen
(Iconography by Pr Mazari).

Depending on its path, the trauma may damage the iris, the lens (post-traumatic cataract and hyphaema) or even the posterior pole (retina and choroid). The extent to which these lesions occur will depend on the strength of the passage of the sharp object through the ocular wall. Functional signs vary: sensation of a foreign body, photophobia, lacrimation, reduced visual acuity, etc.

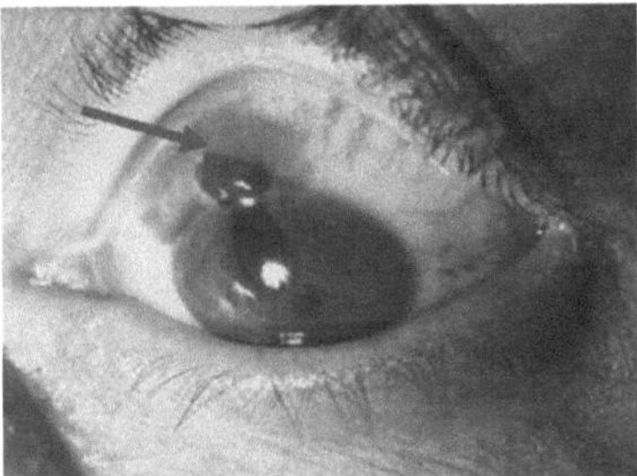

Figure 17: Corneal wound with iris hernia (Iconography by Pr Mazari).

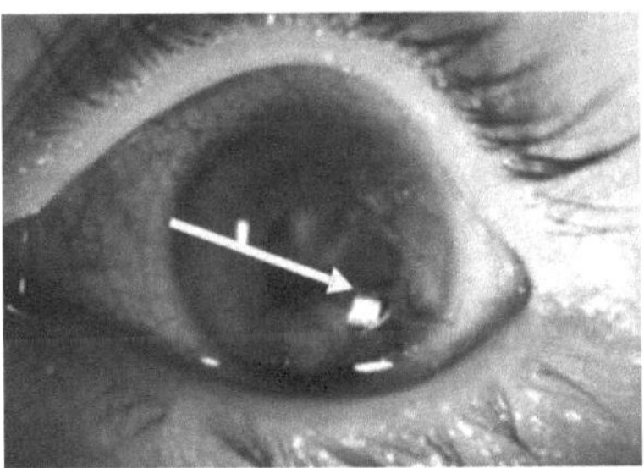

Figure 18: Corneal wound complicated by a ruptured cataract
(Iconography by Pr Mazari).

1-2- Scleral wounds :

They occur when the eye is not in a straight position, i.e. the patient was looking in a given direction at the time of the trauma. The more posterior the impact on the eyeball, the more serious the trauma.

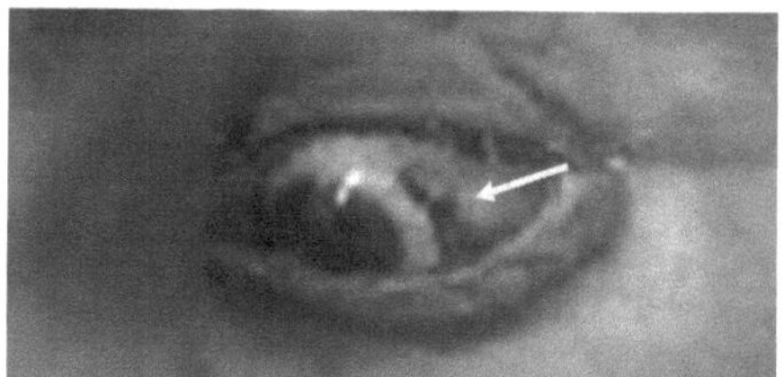

Figure 19: Scleral wound 4mm from the limbus (Iconography by Pr Mazari).

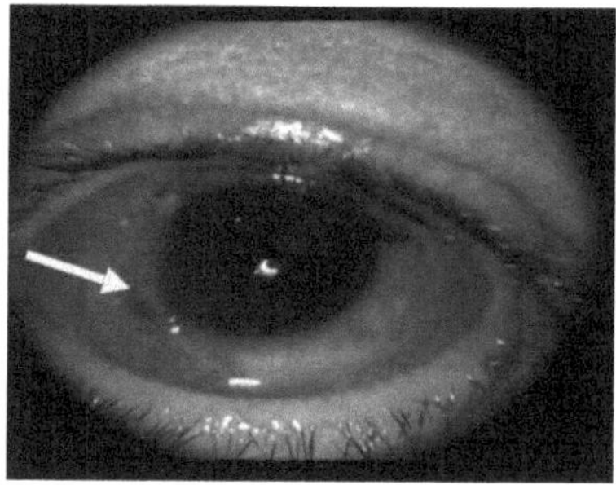

Fig. 20: Sutured para-limbic conjunctivo-scleral wound (Iconography by Pr Mazari).

Treatment :

Certain procedures should be avoided in the event of perforating ocular trauma, namely:
- Instillation of corticosteroid eye drops to reduce the risk of infection.
- Try to open the eye under pressure.

However, you must :

- Apply a non-compressive dressing or shell to protect the eyeball.
- Start the patient on broad-spectrum systemic antibiotics.
- Tetanus prophylaxis for people at risk.

- Request an urgent pre-operative assessment.
- Leave the patient fasting.

Treatment is obviously surgical in a specialised environment under an operating microscope, and consists of trimming the wound and suturing it.

2- Ocular wounds without intraocular foreign bodies :

The foreign body in perforating trauma can be either superficial or deep, with a completely different prognosis.

2-1- Superficial foreign body :

The foreign body is usually small and has low kinetic energy, so the penetrating power is very low. It is generally metal wool used in accidents at work (grinding, sanding). The impact is generally corneal and the prognosis is generally good. There are three possible locations: corneal, in the conjunctival cul de sac and under the upper eyelid, which is why the eyelid must be turned every time the patient consults with a painful red eye suspected of containing a foreign body. A fluorescein test is used to check corneal integrity and the absence of Seidel's sign.

▶   Clinical signs :
The patient consults a few hours to a few days after the trauma for painful red eyes with tearing, photophobia and a sensation of a foreign body.
If the patient does not consult a doctor in time, superinfection can occur, leading to a corneal abscess, which in this case is much more painful.

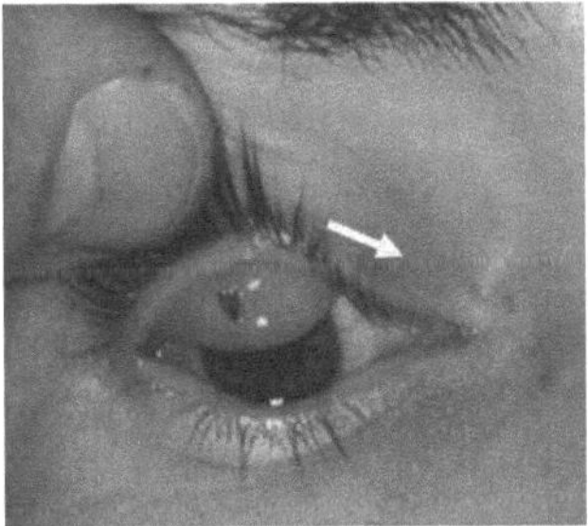

Figure 21: Subpalpebral foreign body.

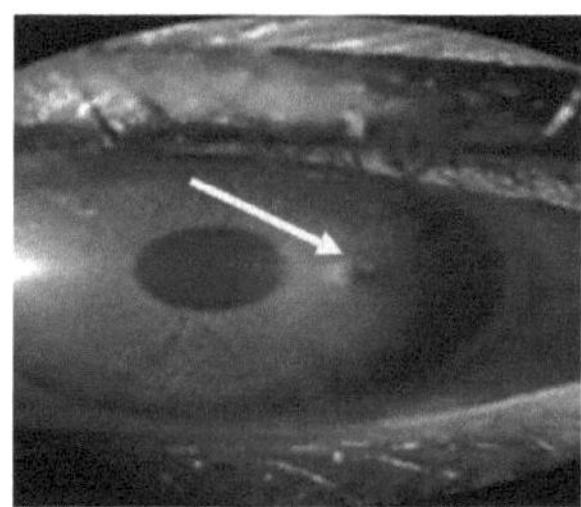

Figure 15: Corneal grit complicated by a corneal abscess (Iconography by Pr Mazari).

▶ Treatment:
- In the absence of superinfection, treatment consists of simple removal of the foreign body using a needle under a slit lamp after a local anaesthetic in eye drops (Novesin), combined with treatment with antibiotics in eye drops and ointment.
- In the event of superinfection: the patient will be admitted to hospital and treated with general and local antibiotics, as well as subconjunctival antibiotics. There is a high risk of the infection spreading inside the eye, leading to endophthalmitis.

2-2- Intraocular foreign body (IOFB) :

Evocative signs :
- It is through questioning that we can first suspect the possibility of an intraocular foreign body. This would be the projection of an iron foreign body by a hammer during DIY, or when working on a metal part (16).
- Certain clinical signs are also suggestive: visible, often punctiform, corneal or scleral portal of entry (remember to look for it by careful clinical examination in the event of subconjunctival haemorrhage), visible path of penetration: lens and/or iris perforation.

Additional tests:In the event of any suspicion of an intraocular foreign body, further diagnostic examinations should be carried out(13)(17) :

*X-rays of the orbit: front, side and Blondeau angle; these will confirm the presence of an oculo-orbital foreign body.
They constitute a forensic document.
*B ultrasound: this enables the foreign body to be located precisely and

confirms its intraocular location; it can also be used to visualise non-radiopaque foreign bodies (non-metallic foreign bodies).

*CT scan: used to locate foreign bodies, in particular if we does not have an ocular B ultrasound;*Magnetic resonance imaging (MRI) is contraindicated because of the risk of mobilising a magnetisable foreign body during the examination.

Early complications of intraocular foreign bodies :

■ Endophthalmitis (intraocular infection): a very serious complication, which can lead to complete blindness.
■ Retinal detachment (RD), whose prognosis is less severe, may be reserved.
■ Traumatic cataracts, the prognosis of which can be favourable with a surgical treatment in the absence of associated lesions

Late complications :
■ Sympathetic ophthalmia: This is a severe autoimmune uveitis of the contralateral eye, occurring from a few weeks to several years after the trauma, the prognosis can be poor.
■ Siderosis and chalcosis: Very severe toxic retinal damage occurring several years after an iron (siderosis) or copper (chalcosis) CEIO: the latter is typically accompanied by a corneal ring called the Kayser-Fleisher ring, identical to that seen in Wilson's disease.)

Treatment :
Given the early or late complications that a foreign body can cause, it must be removed in a specialised environment. An electromagnet can be useful in the case of a metallic foreign body, but in the case of glass, the latter is well tolerated and can therefore be removed at a later date(6).

2-3- Retinal detachment and perforating trauma :
The role of ocular trauma in the causes of retinal detachment is often underestimated compared to other causes such as myopia. For a long time, there was no consensus on the factors that predict the occurrence of retinal detachment following oculo- orbital trauma (7)(8). They are

considered to have a poor prognosis from the outset because of the very marked vitreoretinal proliferation, especially when a foreign body is involved.

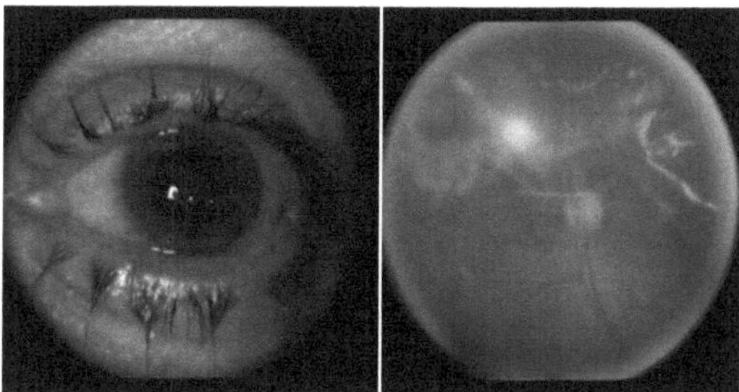

Figure 22: Post-traumatic perforating retinal detachment with intraocular foreign body and persistence of intense fibrosis despite treatment with vitrectomy (Iconography by Pr Mazari).

The main risk factors for retinal detachment depend on the severity of the initial lesions and the pathophysiological mechanisms of the retinovitreal tears and traction involved. Treatment mainly involves endocular surgery(18) to remove retinovitreal traction and apply an endocular tamponade.

D- Chemical and physical burns :

Burns require early treatment. They are most often chemical in nature. Apart from their severity, base burns are the most serious.

▶ Circumstances of occurrence :
1. Industrial accidents: burns resulting from industrial accidents are often serious, because they involve concentrated products (seriousness of base burns +++), or are associated with other traumatic injuries, in the event of an explosion (blast).

2. Domestic accidents: are often related to detergents and are less serious than industrial accidents.

3. Assaults: constitute a significant proportion of chemical eye burns in certain communities, often perpetrated with concentrated alkaline

products and therefore potentially serious.

▶ Burns caused by chemical agents:

▪ Acid burns:
- Acid burn is proportional to the degree of acidity of the product, the lesions are maximal from the outset and are not progressive, which is why they have a better prognosis.
- The product most often incriminated is bleach in the case of domestic trauma.

▪ Alkaline burns:
- Base burns are the most serious. The caustic's action on the surface is more gradual and much more serious, as it penetrates the cornea, passes through it and spreads into the intraocular environment.
- They react with fatty acids (saponification), destroying cell membranes and allowing them to penetrate underlying tissues very quickly.
- The alkaline best known for its severity and rapid penetration is ammonia. Other products frequently found are salt spirit and lime for domestic use.
- If there is any doubt about whether the product in question is acidic or basic, after washing (+++) it is sometimes useful to use pH strips (usually used for urine) to determine the pH of the tears.

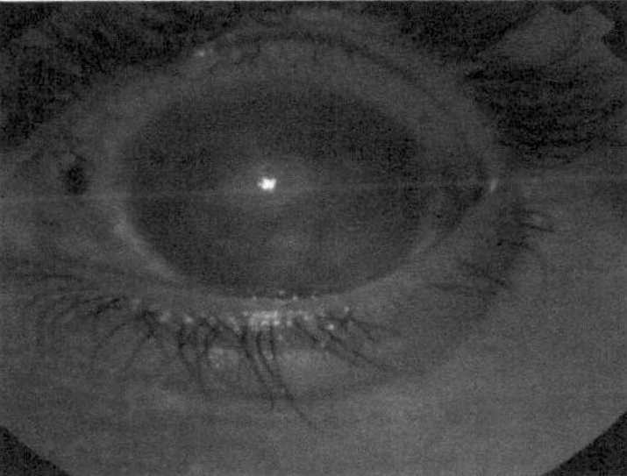

Figure 23: After-effects of a caustic burn caused by an alkaline agent.

Emergency treatment of chemical burns :

- Treatment is instituted immediately +++, at the scene of the accident. Abundant and prolonged washing of the ocular surface with physiological serum (or tap water) for 15 minutes, carefully unfolding the conjunctival

sacs. This should be done as soon as possible after the burn. Any caustic still present should be completely removed. It is often necessary to instil an anaesthetic eye drop to allow the eyelids to open properly.
- The severity of the burn will then be assessed according to the Roper-Hall classification.
Treatment with corticosteroid eye drops should be started as soon as possible to limit the intense inflammatory reaction, which is itself a source of complications.

UV radiation burns:

They are not uncommon (welding, exposure to the sun without eye protection) and are responsible for superficial keratitis. Sometimes the damage is more severe, causing retinal macular photo-trauma.

CONCLUSION

Ocular trauma is a frequent and serious pathology (reserved anatomical and functional prognosis) despite improvements in treatment. The patients who suffer these injuries are young people in the midst of socio-professional activity. Many of these injuries could be avoided by simple protective measures. Unfortunately, this attitude is not respected in our professional circles, prompting the parties concerned to develop, improve and above all impose preventive measures. The latest WHO report stresses the need for urgent action in the following areas: Creating a less dangerous environment. Educating the population, with parents and teachers monitoring children's activities. Legislation on accidents in the workplace, road accidents and the manufacture of dangerous toys, and of course immediate treatment of these injuries (early diagnosis, easy access to care).

BIBLIOGRAPHY

1- Bourges J-L. L'urgence et son vocabulaire. In Société Française d'ophtalmologie, Urgences en ophtalmologie.Rapport 2018. Paris (France): Elsevier Mason; 2018. p. 41- 43.

2- Catalano RA. Ocular emergencies. Philadelphia: WB Saunders; 1992.

3- Bourges JL. Ophthalmological emergencies in French university hospital centres. J Fr Ophtalmol. 2018 ;41(3):218-223

4- Channa R, Zafar SN, Canner JK, Haring RS, Schneider EB, Friedman DS. Epidemiology of Eye-Related Emergency Department Visits. JAMA Ophthalmol. 2016 Mar;134(3):312-9 5- Vartsakis G, Fahy G. The profile of patients attending a triaged eye emergency service. Ir J Med Sci. 2014 Dec;183(4):625-8

6- Odoulami Yehouessi L, Assavedo A, Nkok H, Tchabi S, Doutetien C. Ophthalmological emergencies in hospitals in Borgou. Rev. Afr. Anesth. Med. Urgence 2014; 19 :23-26

7- Mac Ewen C.J, Baines PS, Desai P, Eye injuries in children: the current picture. Br J ophthalmol 1999, 83: 933-936.

8- NEGREL A.D; THYLEFORS . The global impact of eye injuries, ophthalmic Epidemiol, 1998, 5 :143-69

9- Frau E. Traumatismes par contusion du globe oculaire. Encycl Méd Chir (Elsevier, Paris), Ophthalmology 21-700-A-65, 1996, 8p.

10- BEBY F, kodjikian I , ROCHE O. Perforating ocular trauma in children, study retrospective of 57 cases. J Fr ophtalmol, 2OO6, 29: 20-23

11- Lopez meimony M, Miguel Bouras et al ; Urgences ophtalmologiques au travail ; Ophtalmologie 1996 ; 10 :418-21.

12- khalil A, Riss JM, Ridigs B; Intraocular foreign bodies in 27 cases.

13- Cabanis EA, Bourgeois H, Iba-Zizen MT, imagerie en ophtalmologie, Soc Fr opht, edission Masson Paris 1996.

14- Thompson CG, Kumar N, The aetiology of perforating ocular injuries in children. Br J Ophthalmol, 2002, 86:920-922.

15- Faraj, Sayed; Bathen, Marianne Etzelmüller;. All. Published September 1, 2022. Volume 27. Article 101596. © 2022.

16- Kuhn F, et al. The Ocular Trauma Score (OTS). Ophthalmol Clin North Am. 2002; 15:163-5. vi. [PubMed: 12229231]

17- Weichel ED, Colyer MH, Ludlow SE, et al. Combat ocular trauma visual outcome During Operations Iraqi and Enduring Freedom. Ophthalmology. 2008; 115:2235-45. [PubMed: 19041478).

18- Andreoli MT, Andreoli CM. Surgical rehabilitation of the open globe injury patient. Am J Ophthalmol. 2012; 153:856-60. [PubMed: 22265150]

KERATITIS INFECTIOUS

Introduction :

Corneal opacities, which are largely caused by infectious keratitis, are the fourth leading cause of blindness worldwide and are responsible for 10% of avoidable visual impairment in the world's least developed countries(1). In this chapter, we will focus on the main infectious, bacterial, viral and parasitic keratitis encountered in our daily practice.

1- Bacterial keratitis :

Bacterial keratitis is an infection of the cornea caused by one or more bacteria. Clinically, it is characterised by a zone of corneal infiltration underlying an epithelial ulcer, of infectious origin, and leads to tissue damage secondary to an inflammatory reaction(2). Numerous aerobic and anaerobic bacteria are involved in bacterial keratitis of the cornea. However, literature reviews agree that four groups predominate and are involved in 90% of bacterial infections: staphylococci, streptococci, Pseudomonas and enterobacteria (Klebsiella, Enterobacter, Serratia, Moraxella, Proteus)(2,3,4,5). Among these, the main germs responsible are : Staphylococcus aureus, Streptococcus pneumoniae, Pseudomonas aeruginosa and Moraxella.(5) These bacteria obviously correspond mainly to the germs of the ocular commensal flora in its appendages or neighbouring organs (conjunctival, palpebral, cutaneous and nasal flora). However, Gram-negative bacteria from the intestinal and oropharyngeal flora can also be responsible for bacterial keratitis, generally linked to a lack of hygiene. They are particularly common in corneal lesions of contact lens wearers, hospital patients, burn victims and patients on respiratory assistance, especially Pseudomonas aeroginosa, which is specifically linked to the wearing of soft lenses (6,7).

The presence of an altered ocular surface and corneal epithelium is essentially one of the essential conditions for bacterial development within the cornea.

However, there are a few germs that can exceptionally infect the cornea without prior injury thanks to the secretion of proteases that allow intracellular penetration: Neisseria gonorrheae, Neisseria meningitidis, Corynebacterium diphteriae, Haemophilus influenzae biogroup aegyptius, Shigella, Listeria.

Ocular surface defence system :
The ocular surface defence system represented by the eyelids, the tear film and the lacrimal ducts, the corneal epithelium and its innervation, the conjunctival immune tissue and the palpebral and conjunctival bacterial flora play a vital role in protecting the cornea against microbial aggression. The occurrence of isolated bacterial keratitis generally suggests that certain ocular surface defence systems must be deficient, allowing germs to penetrate and proliferate in the cornea (2).

Risk factors :
The risk factors for bacterial keratitis vary according to geographical, social and age factors (8) . The most important risk factors include wearing contact lenses, corneal (refractive) surgery and eye trauma. In elderly patients, chronic ocular surface pathologies (dry eye, bullous dystrophy, neurotrophic keratitis, fibrosing conjunctivitis, neuroparalytic conjunctivitis, trachoma, limbal stem cell deficiency) and palpebral anomalies are often implicated in bacterial keratitis(8,9). Other risk factors were found in the case series: immunodepression (diabetes, corticosteroids, human immunodeficiency virus HIV, alcoholism, malnutrition), self-medication, prolonged prescription of eye drops (corticosteroids, long-term antibiotics). However, current studies place the wearing of contact lenses as the main risk factor for serious bacterial keratitis, increased by night-time or prolonged wear. Or in cases of underlying corneal pathology or poor hygiene(17-18).

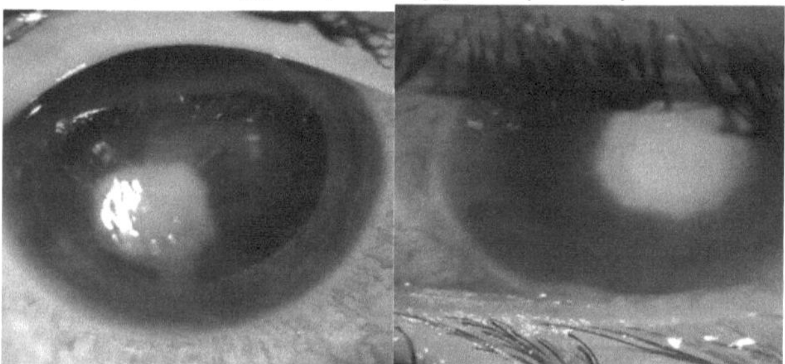

ab

Figure 1: (a and b) Bilateral Staphylococcus aureus abscess in a contact lens wearer. (Iconography by Pr F Mazari).

Clinical diagnosis :

The clinical signs of infectious keratitis include aspecific symptoms that often appear abruptly, such as pain exacerbated by blinking of the eyelids, ocular redness, photophobia and blepharospasm. The reduction in visual acuity depends on the location of the infection in relation to the visual axis, The clinical signs that guide the diagnosis in favour of infectious keratitis include the presence of fluorescein-taking corneal ulceration accompanied by a diffuse (keratitis) or localised (abscess) stromal infiltrate, and suppurative stromal inflammation that may be diffuse, focal, multifocal or marginal. Inflammation of the anterior chamber can be seen in the presence of a Tyndall or hypopyon. The severity criteria are listed in the table below:

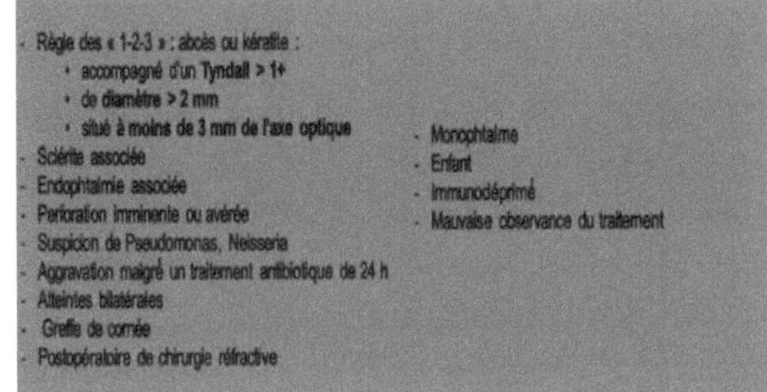

Table 1: Severity criteria for bacterial keratitis*.

Most of these criteria also represent the criteria that require hospitalisation
Note that specific characteristics may be indicative of certain bacteria involved:

- Gram-positive cocci cause round, grey-white abscesses (localised stromal infiltration) with clean margins. Staphylococci are naturally present in the normal bacterial flora, and cause infectious keratitis mainly in cases of pathological cornea (dry eye, bullous keratitis, herpes) or risk factors such as contact lens wear, diabetes and advanced age.

- Streptococcus pneumoniae appears in cases of corneal trauma or filtering surgery. Pneumococcal abscesses progress rapidly and reach the deep stroma, with a large abscess associated with radiations along Descemet's membrane, a hypopyon, endothelial fibrin deposits and may progress to perforation.

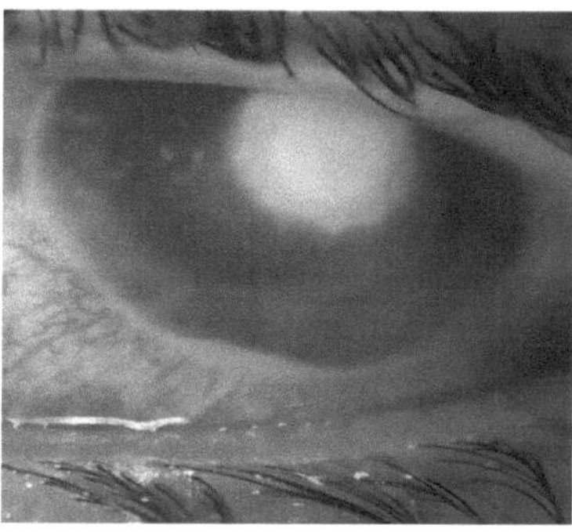

Figure 2: Bacterial keratitis (Pseudomonas aeruginosa). Presence o f a slide (Iconography by Pr F Mazari).

- Staphylococcus aureus causes rapidly progressive infiltration associated with moderate inflammation of the anterior chamber.

However, bacteriological analysis by **corneal scraping** remains the reference **sample**, enabling a precise diagnosis to be made of the bacteria involved. **An antibiotic susceptibility test is** systematically carried out and delivered within 48 to 72 hours with a view to appropriate treatment.

Practical management :

Bacterial keratitis is a real therapeutic emergency, and timely, appropriate treatment is the rule in order to avoid the dreaded complications of bacterial keratitis, such as corneal perforation, endophthalmitis and permanent corneal opacity(19). It should be remembered that a corneal abscess or keratitis with an infectious appearance is bacterial until proven otherwise.

The general consensus i s that before any treatment with probabilistic antibiotic therapy is started, it is essential to take a sample of secretions or from the site of infection for direct analysis, then to culture the germs sampled, and finally to perform an antibiogram in order to subsequently adapt the antibiotic therapy.

Unlike infections in other tissues, bacterial keratitis is treated mainly with **topical antibiotics**. Topical treatment is more effective due to the avascular nature of corneal tissue and the presence of the blood-water barrier. These treatments include eye drops, ointments and gels. In superficial ocular infections, topical antibiotic therapy offers equal or greater bioavailability at the ocular surface than systemic antibiotic therapy and can treat most serious ocular surface infections(20, 22) .

However, only around 1% of the active ingredients used reach the anterior chamber of the eye. Therefore, in cases of intraocular damage or infection of the adjacent sclera and gonococcal keratitis, an indication for additional systemic treatment should be established. On the other hand, systemic application has no real benefit in isolated keratitis, as only low concentrations are reached in the cornea (20).

One of the decisive factors in the successful treatment of ulcerative bacterial keratitis is the initial use of high doses of antimicrobial agents.
A loading dose should be administered first, followed by a maintenance dose. The **loading dose** can be administered every 5 minutes for the first two weeks.
hour to reduce the bacterial load as much as possible, and the antibiotic can be administered every hour thereafter for 24 to 48 hours. If eye drops containing preservatives are used, their toxic effects on tissues must be taken into account. (22). The therapeutic strategy is then adapted according to the clinical course and the results of the microbiology. In cases of bacterial keratitis where the results of the antibiogram and culture have not yet been returned, or if no germ is visible or the direct examination is negative, it is preferable to continue with a **broad-spectrum antibiotic treatment**.
Indeed, the rate of false-negative results from bacteriological sampling is fairly high according to the literature: 20 to 30% according to O'Brien(14) and 22% according to McLeod (23).The choice of an antibiotic or combination of antibiotics must include bacteriological, pharmacokinetic and toxicological considerations, and take into account the risk of selecting resistant mutants.(16) The duration of treatment should be at least 15 days.
The eplthellum of the cornea and conjunctiva represents a major obstacle to the penetration of active ingredients by the topical route. Lipophilicity, viscosity and molecular weight are important characteristics of the antibiotic to ensure good penetration and diffusion of the active ingredient through the ocular surface barriers. Molecules such as fluoroquinolones, which have a balanced hydrophilic/lipophilic ratio,

penetrate the anterior chamber topically through the epithelial barrier and systemically through the blood-aqueous barrier(24).Molecular parameters such as reduced viscosity and low molecular weight are thought to favour the penetration of active ingredients into the aqueous humour and other tissues. Vancomycin, for example, has a high molecular weight, which represents an obstacle to the antibiotic's penetration (24).

Practical treatment of bacterial keratitis :

- If there are no signs of seriousness, treatment can be carried out on an outpatient basis. A mono- or bi-therapy based on "classic" antibiotic therapy is generally implemented, with active and close monitoring for 24 hours.
The antibiotics from the class of **fluoroquinolones** (Ofloxacin, Ciprofloxacin) are used as first-line treatment, with or without a combination of antibiotics from another class (**Aminoside, Macrolide or Rifamycin**). If a multi-bacterial infection is suspected, a combination of **cephalosporin and aminoglycoside** is often used as first-line treatment. If an atypical mycobacterial infection is diagnosed (M. fortuitum), a poly-antibiotherapy is prescribed from the outset, giving a quinolone, an aminoglycoside, a tetracycline and a cephalosporin. As already mentioned, a loading dose is given by instilling a drop once every hour for 24 to 48 hours. Antibiotic therapy is then adapted according to the clinical response and the results of additional microbiological tests.

- In the presence of signs of seriousness, hospitalisation is the rule and a combination of antibiotics will be rapidly introduced depending on the results of the antibiogram. On the other hand, if the bacteriological examination is negative, broad-spectrum antibiotic therapy is recommended to target both gram-positive cocci and gram-negative bacilli, for example the combination of: Ticarcillin (7mg/ml) + Gentamicin (15 mg/ml) + Vancomycin (50 mg/ml) with the same instillation protocol as above.
Some antibiotics, such as cefuroxime, can be administered by intrastromal injection into the infected area every 48 to 72 hours. hours, in order to increase their local concentration while reducing their toxicity

on the ocular surface.

The favourable clinical course is marked by re-epithelialisation of the injured area and a reduction in the infiltrated area.
In all cases, if antibiotic therapy is effective, the progression of keratitis is normally halted within 48 to 72 hours.

If there is no therapeutic response or if the condition worsens, the use of fortified eye drops after corneal sampling is recommended.

Topical fortified antibiotics are medicines prepared in the hospital from antibiotics marketed in powder, lyophilisate or injectable form. These antibiotics have two major advantages: they contain a high concentration of the active ingredient and give us a wider choice of antibiotics.Their disadvantage lies in the risk of toxicity secondary to their formulation (acid pH, relative hyper osmolarity). And their short shelf life. The best-tolerated eye drops are those based on Ceftazidime and Cefazolin.Other antibiotics can be used in the form of fortified eye drops:

•Beta-lactams: penems (penicillin, carboxypenicillin), penemes (carbapenems) and cephemes (cephalosporins).
•Glycopeptides: Vancomycin is an antibiotic in the glycopeptide class.

Adjuvant measures to antibiotic therapy :

- stop wearing contact lenses and take strict hygiene measures.
- Contraindication of corticosteroid therapy.
- The treatment of chronic pathologies of the corneal surface as well as management of any systemic disease.

Most cases of bacterial keratitis resolve with medical treatment if they are treated early, and a microbiological examination is carried out if necessary. Appropriate treatment to control risk factors and treat aetiological causes can improve prognosis. Finally, patient education and information Contact lens wearers play an important role in preventing bacterial infections.

2- Amebic keratitis :

They are considered rare and serious infections, threatening visual and anatomical prognosis. Its incidence has risen sharply in tandem with contact lens wear, which remains the main risk factor.

Amoebae are **unicellular eukaryotes** from the large **protozoan** family that carry out their entire cycle **in nature and do not require a host**. Free-living amoebae are ubiquitous in the natural environment, unlike parasitic (or intestinal) amoebae, which live in the digestive tract of animals. They are found in the air, soil and water (taps, swimming pools, reservoirs, cisterns, sewers, air conditioning and humidification systems, the sea, ponds, rivers, lakes, etc.). They are able to move in "amoeboid" movements thanks to the pseudopods on their surface. They feed mainly on micro-organisms through phagocytosis (25).

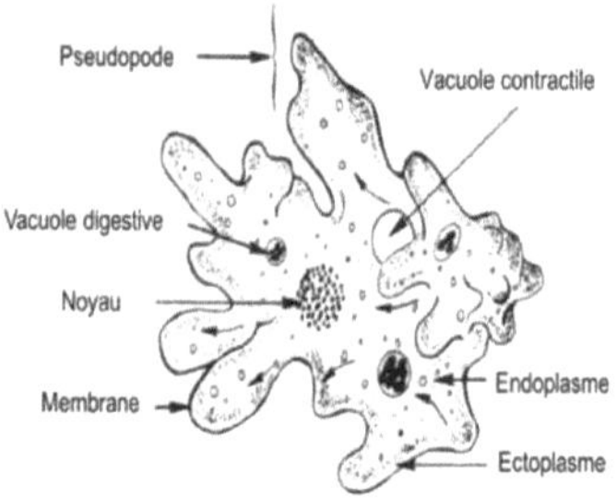

Figure 3: Cellular organisation of an amoeba.

The amoeba Acanthamoeba is the pathogen most frequently found in infectious keratitis. Acanthamoeba keratitis is contracted by direct contact with a pathological and previously injured cornea. It is notoriously devastating due to its ability to adhere to epithelial cells and produce proteases, peroxidases and other proteins that destroy the extracellular matrix and tissues(26).

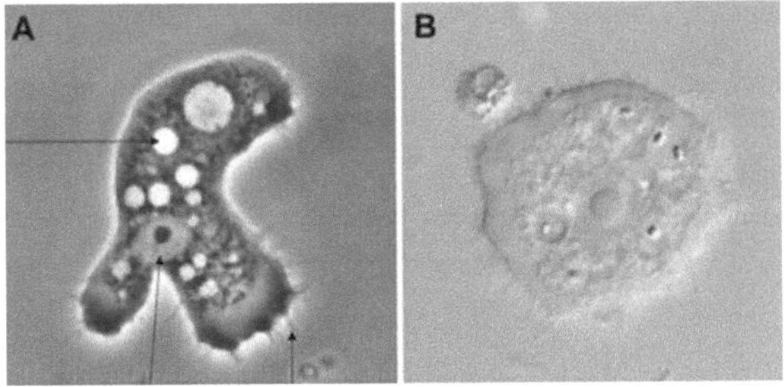

Figure 4: Acanthamoeba trophozoites (A) phase contrast, (B) brightfield microscopy (Iconography reviewed In the lIterature).

Thinking about this is the most important step in diagnosing AK . As a general rule, amoebic keratitis should be considered in all contact lens wearers and in all cases of corneal trauma involving exposure to contaminated soil or water. Symptoms are often **unilateral**, and exceptionally bilateral. Amebic keratitis progresses **slowly** from the epithelium to the corneal stroma. Clinical symptoms include photophobia, massive pain, tears and ocular irritation. Corneal lesions caused by Acanthamoeba are highly polymorphic, and can be summarised in the table below according to the stage of amoebic keratitis.

Stadium at the amoebic keratitis	Clinical signs
Early Amoebic Keratitis The first four to six weeks of infection Corneal lesions predominantly at epithelial and subepithelial level	Superficial punctate keratitis Irregularity of the epithelial surface (lines or ulcers, gelatinous appearance) Epithelial microcysts Pseudodendrites Diffuse or focal epithelial or subepithelial infiltrates Keratoneuritis
Late Amoebic Keratitis After four to six weeks Mainly stromal disease	Persistent or recurrent Persistent or recurrent epithelial ulceration(s) Disciform stromal infiltrate Immune ring (annular infiltrate) Satellite lesions Cast iron Slimming Descemetocele Perforation Neovascularisation Scleritis Uveitis, hypopyon Cataract Hypertonia Hypotonia Choroiditis Endophthalmitis Retinal detachment Optic neuritis Pthyse

Table 2: Clinical manifestations of amebic keratitis.

Indeed, in the early stages, KA can easily be confused with herpes simplex keratitis, while in the advanced stages, the infection resembles the clinical image of fungal keratitis or a corneal ulcer. The only pathognomonic clinical sign of AK is radial keratoneuritis, which is however inconstant and only found in 15 to 20% of cases (27).

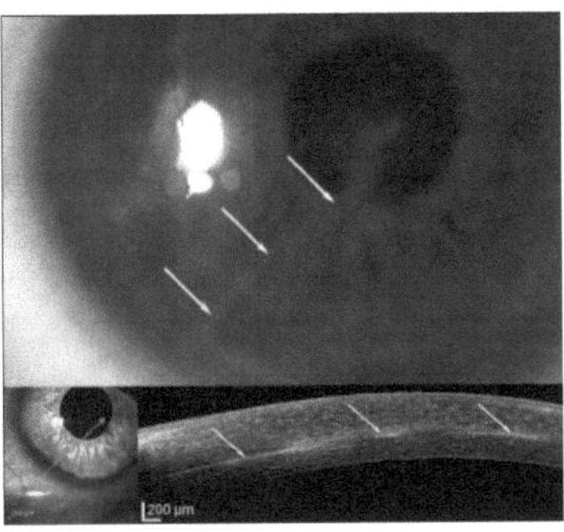

Figure 5:Amebic keratitis in a contact lens wearer, which had been progressing for 2 weeks. Note the radial keratoneuritis (arrows): this corresponds to infiltration of the corneal nerves by inflammatory cells and explains the intensity of the ocular pain felt by the patient. Corresponding aspect on OCT-SD corneal module (Iconography SFO report).

As a result, the diagnosis of amoebic keratitis is rarely made as a first line of defence, and topical antibiotic and antiviral treatments are often introduced, leading to therapeutic failures and clinical worsening. Indeed, if diagnosis and treatment are delayed, the parasite penetrates deep into the corneal stroma and successful therapy becomes very complicated. When the parasite reaches the stroma, there are significant inflammatory reactions, a large epithelial ulcer and the stroma may take the form of localised or diffuse infiltrates. It can also lead to complications (28).

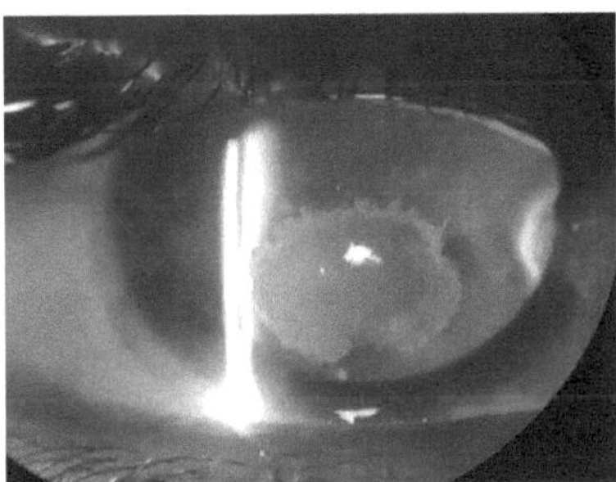

Figure 6: Advanced amoebic keratitis affecting the stroma in a patient wearing contact lenses. (Iconography by Pr F Mazari).

Direct detection of the causal agent in the sample by corneal scraping is the only reliable diagnostic method with certainty. The corneal sample should be taken after abundant washing of the conjunctival cul-de-sacs with sterile physiological saline, without any treatment or after a therapeutic window of 24 to 48 hours. Amoebae should also be looked for in the lenses, the case or the maintenance solution (28,29).

Management of amoebic keratitis :

Early diagnosis and appropriate treatment have improved the quality of life of patients. The prognosis for this condition was long considered fatal. Certain steps can help with amoebic treatment. These include early epithelial debridement to eliminate the majority of amoebae. To date, no single effective treatment has been described for Acanthamoeba infection, regardless of the genotype that causes it. It is difficult to establish a single treatment regimen due to the small number of cases reported, the pathogenic variability of different strains and the intrinsically fluctuating nature of the disease process (27). It is applied after corneal samples have been taken, on the basis of a clinical diagnosis. The microbiological results then confirm the diagnosis.Management is primarily medical, and in the event of failure, treatment can be administered. can be maintained.As there is no consensus on treatment, the medical protocol is empirical.

Amebic keratitis is a therapeutic emergency and hospitalisation is recommended.Biguanides (Chlorhexidine (0.02% and 0.2%), polyhexamethylene biguanide (pHMB) (0.02% and 0.06%) and topical diamidines are the treatments with the most significant and effective cysticide and antitrophozoite activity. The mode of action of these two molecules is not clearly elucidated. They are hospital preparations.

a. Biguanides :

Biguanides are cationic disinfectants, including PHMB and CLX. The first case of KA treated with PHMB was described in 1992 (30). The first clinical use of chlorhexidine eye drops was described in 1994 (31) act on both trophozoite and cystic forms by altering the cytoplasmic membrane of amoebae and inducing cell lysis for CLX and apoptosis for PHMB.In current practice, biguanide eye drops are used at a concentration of 0.02%, i.e. 200 µg/mL, with satisfactory clinical efficacy. A dose of one drop every hour, including at night for 48 to 72 hours, which requires hospitalisation. To minimise toxicity, eye drops are administered 4 times a day for several months, until the cystic and trophozoite forms of Acanthamoeba are eliminated. There is no definite consensus on the duration of treatment, which often lasts more than 6 months, or even 1 year in some cases(32,33).

b. Diamines :
Propamidine 0.1% (i.e. 1mg/mL) and hexamidine 0.1% have antibacterial properties, but their mechanism remains unknown, as does Désomédine®.
One study showed hexamidine to be more effective in vitro than propamidine, which was somewhat toxic(34,35).

c- Local corticosteroid therapy :
Topical corticosteroids can be effective in cases of intense pain or corneal ulcers, but it is recommended to wait 2 weeks of effective treatment with biguanide before administering them. This allows as many trophozoites and cystic forms as possible to be eliminated. Prednisolone 0.5% is given 4 times a day or dexamethasone 0.1% at variable intervals depending on clinical signs (25,26).

3- **Herpetic keratitis :**
Ocular herpes simplex virus-1 (HSV-1) is thought to affect 90,000 people in France, and the risk of developing it is around 1% over the course of a human lifetime. It can affect all the main ocular tissues (eyelids, conjunctiva, cornea, uveal tract and retina), giving rise to a clinical polymorphism. The most common presentation is epithelial or dendritic keratitis(37). Deep stromal damage is the most serious form of damage, leading to corneal opacification and loss of vision.

Herpes simplex virus type 1 is a strictly human virus and is transmitted by direct contact. It is found in eye infections in adults and children, while type 2 is mainly responsible for maternal-foetal contamination during vaginal delivery. The immediate risk is neurological damage leading to meningoencephalitis seven days after birth, and the longer-term risk is the development of necrotising retinitis(38,39). Recent studies show HSV-1 seroprevalence of over 50% and between 75% and 90% in general adult populations in the United States, Germany and Tanzania respectively (40,41). The majority of the population has already been infected with the HSV-1 virus and probably carries a latent viral load. In fact, 95% of primary HSV-1 infections are asymptomatic, and symptomatic ocular forms are rare because they generally affect the oropharyngeal sphere.Dendritic epithelial lesions are thought to be the most common type of recurrent keratitis (56.3%), followed by herpetic stromal keratitis (29.5%) and geographic epithelial lesions (9.8%)(42).

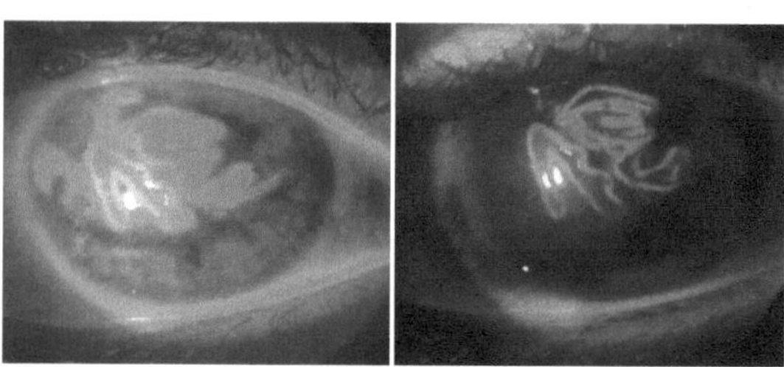

Figure 7: Map-like ulcer in a patient with recurrent herpetic keratitis.
(Iconography by Pr F Mazari).

In the Herpetic Eye Disease Study, stromal herpetic keratitis due to HSV-1 (HSK) accounted for 44% of recurrences, representing a significant problem in ocular infection. (43,44)
In the literature, three categories of the population appear to be at risk of developing particularly symptomatic forms: children are very rarely affected, but develop more severe, bilateral and recurrences compared with adults(45,46), atopic patients whose ocular herpes takes a more severe form than the general population (necrotic forms of stromal keratitis)(47), and finally diabetic patients have a higher than average incidence of first infection and recurrence(46).

Contamination occurs mainly through saliva
The HSV-1 virus replicates in the epithelium of the site of primary infection (mainly in the oropharyngeal tract) and spreads through the nerve endings by retrograde axonal transport into the nervous system, where it lies dormant, mostly in asymptomatic form. The main site of latency for the virus is Gasser's trigeminal ganglion, a relay of the sensory nerve pathways of the face. Over 90% of the population over the age of 60 has a latent herpes infection in the nervous system. Because of this latent state, HSV is present throughout the life of the infected host.

Reactivation of the virus' replicative cycle is triggered by physical or biological factors via stimulation of transcription factors. Physical factors that stimulate or injure the corneal nerves, such as eye surgery, ultraviolet radiation and cold, are formidable risk factors that stimulate viral replication. The same applies to chemical factors such as prostaglandins secreted during an inflammatory reaction, alpha-adrenergics or corticoids, which have a promoting effect on the synthesis of certain transcription factors and are therefore direct activators of viral replication.

Management of herpetic keratitis :

Ocular herpes is a potentially serious condition that can also lead to permanent loss of visual acuity if not treated properly.Current herpes antivirals active against HSV viruses have a virostatic role that limits the replication phase of the virus. They are not active in the latency phase, which makes it impossible to eradicate the virus, hence the recurrence of herpes pathology.

We have :

- Two systemic antivirals (aciclovir orally and intravenously, and valaciclovir orally).
- Three topical therapies (aciclovir ointment, trifluridine eye drops and ganciclovir gel).

Aciclovir is the treatment of choice for HSV infections. It is available in oral form as tablets and a drinkable suspension, as an intravenous injection, and as a topical ointment containing 3%. In the case of the ointment, vision is impaired after application, but it is very well tolerated. The oral doses of aciclovir and valaciclovir for ocular herpes are 2g in five doses and 1g in two doses respectively.

At this dose of 2g/day, oral aciclovir produces an "effective" antiviral concentration in tears, i.e. greater than that which inhibits replication of 50% of viral particles.

As preventive cover, for aciclovir and valaciclovir are 800mg in two doses versus 500mg in one dose.Ganciclovir (GCV) is available as a topical ophthalmic gel containing 0.15%.

Adjuvant treatments :

Corticosteroids :
Inflammation is the main cause of visual loss due to HSV infection of the eye, hence the need to combine corticoids with antivirals once viral replication has been inhibited and controlled with antivirals, and once the lesions have stabilised. Corticosteroids are formally contraindicated in the case of pure epithelial keratitis (dendritic type), or necrotic stromal keratitis, at the risk of aggravating the lesions and progressing towards corneal melting. The HEDS studies confirmed that topical corticosteroid therapy reduced the progression or persistence of HSV-related inflammation compared with placebo by 68%(48,49).Monitoring must be rigorous and weaning must be gradual in order to avoid a rebound effect It is important to continue antiviral therapy for one month afterwards. initiation of corticosteroid therapy.Therapeutic indications: in practice, depending on the degree of severity, the topical form in eye drops or ointment is used for herpetic infections without signs of severity, the oral form is administered for severe infections, and the systemic form by intravenous injection may be used for a few days when the oral route is inaccessible or the inflammation is very severe, with oral relay (50,51).

CONCLUSION

At the end of this presentation, it is clear that infectious keratitis is a complex, multifactorial condition requiring adequate clinical knowledge in order to target the pathogen in question. Biological tests are still essential in current practice for rapid diagnosis. Despite appropriate antimicrobial treatments for most of the pathogens involved in infectious keratitis, and the considerable improvement in antimicrobial treatments over time, clinical results often remain mediocre or even ineffective.

BIBLIOGRAPHY

1. Austin A, Lietman T, Rose-Nussbaumer J. Update on the Management of Infectious Keratitis. Ophthalmology. nov 2017;124(11):1678-89.
2. Austin A, Lietman T, Rose-Nussbaumer J. Update on the Management of Infectious Keratitis. Ophthalmology. nov 2017;124(11):1678-89.
3. Tabbara KF, Bou Chacra CT. Infectious keratitis. In: Tabbara KF, Abu El- Asrar AM, Khairallah M, editors. Ocular Infections. New York, NY: Springer Berlin Heidelberg; 2014:73-94.
4. Rachwalik D, Pleyer U. Bakterielle Keratitis. Klin Monatsblätter Für Augenheilkd. 17 June 2015;232(06):738-44.
5. Bourcier T, Chaumeil C. Bacterial keratitis. In: Bourcier T, Chaumeil C, Bor- derie V et al. Corneal infections. Diagnosis and treatment. Paris: Elsevier; 2004, p. 39-63.
6. Ancele E, Lequeux L, Fournie P, et al. Severe bacterial keratitis. A clinical, epidemio- logic, and microbiologic study. J Fr Ophthalmol 2009; 32: 558-65.
7. Green M, Apel A, Stapleton F. Risk factors and causative organisms in microbial keratitis. Cornea 2008; 27: 22-7.
8. Sandali O, Gaujoux T, Goldschmidt P, et al. Infectious keratitis in severe limbal stem cell deficiency: characteristics and risk factors. Ocul Immunol Inflamm 2012 ; 20 : 182-9.
9. Jhanji V, Constantinou M, Taylor HR, Vajpayee RB. Microbiological and clinical profile of patients with microbial keratitis residing in nursing homes. Br J Ophthalmol 2009; 93: 1639-42.
10. Yildiz EH, Airiani S, Hammersmith KM et al. Trends in contact lens-related corneal ulcers at a tertiary referral centre. Cornea 2012; 31: 1097-1102.
11. Stapleton F, Keay L, Edwards K et al. The incidence of contact lens-related microbial keratitis in Australia. Ophthalmology 2008; 115: 1655-1662.
12. Eye drops and other topical antibiotics for superficial eye infections. Argumentaire. Médecine Mal Infect. Dec 2004;34(12):612-27.
13. Lin A, Rhee MK, Akpek EK, et al. Bacterial keratitis preferred p Ophthalmology. 2019;126:P1-P55. doi:10.1016/ j.ophtha.2018.10.018.
14. O'Brien TP. Bacterial keratitis. in Krachmer, Mannis, Holland: The cornea. Mosby, Saint-Louis, 1997;94:1139-89.
15. McLeod SD, Kolahdouz-Isfahani A, Rostamian K, Flowers CW, Lee PP, McDonnell PJ. The role of smears, cultures, and antibiotic sensitivity testing in the management of suspected infectious keratitis. Ophthalmology 1996;103:23-8.
16. Robert P-Y, Adenis J-P. Bacterial keratitis.

/data/revues/01815512/00220010/1104/ [Internet]. 8 March 2008 [cited 16 June 2020]; Available from: https://www.em-consulte.com/en/article/111129

17. Bourcier T, Sauer A, Saleh M, Dory A, Prévost G, Labetoulle M. Bacterial keratitis. Datatraitesop21-63295 [Internet]. 30 Oct 2013 [cited 8 May 2020]; Available from: https://www.em-consulte.com/en/article/846707

18. Le Grand Y. Optique physiologique. Paris: Édition de la revue d'optique; 1956.

19. Maurice D. The structure and transparency of the cornea. J Phisiol 1957;136:263-86.

20. Dahlgren MA, Lingappan A, Wilhelmus KR. The clinical diagnosis of microbial keratitis. Am J Ophthalmol 2007; 143: 940-4.

21. Gritz DC, Kwitko S, Trousdale MD, Gonzalez VH, McDonnell PJ. Recurrence of microbial keratitis concomitant with antiinflammatory treatment in an animal model. Cornea. Sep; 1992

22. Tomas-Barberan S, Fagerholm P. Influence of topical treatment on epithelial woundhealing and pain in the early postoperative period following photorefractive keratectomy. Acta ophthalmologica Scandinavica. Apr; 1999 77(2):135-138. 11(5):404-408

(23). Ly CN, Pham JN, Badenoch PR, Bell SM, Hawkins G, Rafferty DL, et al. Bacteria commonly isolated from keratitis specimens retain antibiotic susceptibility to fluoroquinolones and gentamicin plus cephalothin. Clin Experiment Ophthalmol, 2006;34:44-50.

24. Hyndiuk RA, Eiferman RA, Caldwell DR, Rosenwasser GO, Santos CI, Katz HR, et al. Comparison of ciprofloxacin ophthalmic solution 0.3% to fortified tobramycin-cefazolin in treating bacterial corneal ulcers. Ciprofloxacin Bacterial Keratitis Study Group. Ophthalmology, 1996; 103:1854-62; [discussion 1862-3].

25. McClellan K, Howard K, Niederkorn JY, Alizadeh H. Effect of steroids on Acanthamoeba cysts and trophozoites. Invest Ophthalmol Vis Sci 2001; 42: 2885-93.

26 John T, Lin J, Sahm D, Rockey JH. Effects of corticosteroids in experimental Acanthamoeba keratitis. Rev Infect Dis 1991; 13: S440-442.

27. Chaumeil C, Malet F. Infectious complications. In: Rapport SFO. Les lentilles de contact. Issy- les- Moulineaux: Masson; 2009, p. 873-932.

28. McClellan K, Howard K, Niederkorn JY, Alizadeh H. Effect of steroids on Acanthamoeba cysts and trophozoites. Invest Ophthalmol Vis Sci 2001; 42: 2885-93.172.

29. John T, Lin J, Sahm D, Rockey JH. Effects of corticosteroids in experimental Acanthamoeba keratitis. Rev Infect Dis 1991; 13: S440-442.

30. Larkin DF, Kilvington S, Dart JK. Treatment of Acanthamoeba keratitis with polyhexamethylene biguanide. Ophthalmology. 1992;99(2):185-91.

31. Hay J, Kirkness CM, Seal DV. Drug resistance and Acanthamoeba keratitis: the quest for alternative antiprotozoal chemotherapy. Eye (Lond). 1994;8(5):555-63.

32. Szczotka-Flynn LB, Shovlin JP, Schnider CM, Caffery BE, Alfonso EC, Carnt NA, et al. American Academy of Optometry Microbial Keratitis Think Tank. Optom Vis Sci. 2021;98(3):182-98.

33. Chlorhexidine [Internet]. Available at: https://upload.wikimedia.org/wikipedia/commons/thumb/5/5b/Chlorhexidin e.p ng/1200px-Chlorhexidine.png

34. Murdoch, D.; Gray, T.B.; Cursons, R.; Parr, D. Acanthamoeba Keratitis in New Zealand, Including Two Cases with in Vivo Resistance to Polyhexamethylene Biguanide. Aust N Z J Ophthalmol **1998**, 26, 231-236, doi:10.1111/j.1442-9071.1998.tb01317.x.

35. Tseng, S.H.; Lin, S.C.; Chen, F.K. Is Polyhexamethylene Biguanide Alone Effective for Acanthamoeba Keratitis? Cornea **1998**, 17, 345-346, doi:10.1097/00003226-199805000-00019.

36. Lam, D.S.; Lyon, D.; Poon, A.S.; Rao, S.K.; Fan, D.S. Polyhexamethylene Biguanide (0.02%) Alone Is Not Adequate for Treating Chronic Acanthameoba Keratitis. Eye (Lond) **2000**, 14 (Pt 4), 678-679, doi:10.1038/eye.2000.174.

37. Lobo A-M, Agelidis AM, Shukla D. Pathogenesis of herpes simplex keratitis: the host cell response and ocular surface sequelae to infection and inflammation. Ocul Surf. Jan 2019;17(1):40-9.

38. Farooq AV, Shukla D. Herpes simplex epithelial and stromal keratitis: an epidemiologic update. Surv Ophthalmol 2012;57:448-62.

39. Niessen F. Viral embryofoetopathies. In: Offret H, editor. OEil et virus. Paris: Masson; 2000.

40. Rabenau HF, Buxbaum S, Preiser W, Weber B, Doerr HW. Seroprevalence of herpes simplex virus types 1 and type 2 in the Frankfurt am Main area, Germany. Med Microbiol Immunol. 2002; 190:153-160. [PubMed: 12005327].

41. Xu F, Sternberg MR, Kottiri BJ, McQuillan GM, Lee FK, Nahmias AJ, Berman SM, Markowitz LE. Trends in herpes simplex virus type 1 and type 2 seroprevalence in the United States. Jama. 2006; 296:964-973. [PubMed: 16926356].

42. Masson E. Fungal keratitis [Internet]. EM-Consulte. [cited 19 Oct 2020]. Available from: https://www.em-consulte.com/article/664823/keratites- fungi

43. Mikloska Z, Bosnjak L, Cunningham AL. Immature monocyte-derived dendritic cells are productively infected with herpes simplex virus type 1.

J Virol. 2001; 75:5958-5964.

44. Liesegang TJ. Herpes simplex virus epidemiology and ocular importance. Cornea. 2001; 20:1-13.

45. Chong EM, Wilhelmus KR, Matoba AY, Jones DB, Coats DK, Paysse EA. Herpes simplex virus keratitis in children. Am J Ophthalmol 2004;138:474-5.

46. Kaiserman I, Kaiserman N, Nakar S, Vinker S. Herpetic eye disease in diabetic patients. Ophthalmology 2005;112:2184-8.

47. Rezende RA, Bisol T, Hammersmith K, Hofling-Lima AL, Webster GF, Freitas JF, et al. Epithelial herpetic simplex keratitis recurrence and graft survival after corneal transplantation in patients with and without atopy. Am J Ophthalmol 2007;143:623-8.

48. Wilhelmus KR, Gee L, Hauck WW, et al. Herpetic Eye Disease Study. A controlled trial of topical corticosteroids for herpes simplex stromal keratitis. Ophthalmology. 1994;101(12):1883- 1895; discussion 1895-1886.

49. Frobert E, Burrel S, Ducastelle-Lepretre S, et al. Resistance of herpes simplex viruses to acyclovir: an update from a ten-year survey in France. Antiviral Res. 2014;111:36-41

50, The Herpetic Eye Disease Study Group. Acyclovir for the prevention of recurrent herpes simplex virus eye disease. N Engl J Med 1998;339:300-6.

51. The Herpetic Eye Disease Study Group. Oral acyclovir for herpes simplex virus eye disease: effect on prevention of epithelial keratitis and stromal keratitis. Arch Ophthalmol 2000;118:1030-6.

DACRYOCYSTITIS

INTRODUCTION :

Dacryocystitis is an infectious inflammation of the lacrimal sac, caused by intra-sacular stasis of tears following obstruction of the vertical portion of the lacrimal ducts, most commonly the nasolacrimal duct. It is a fairly common pathology in routine ophthalmological practice (1,2).

CLINICAL MANIFESTATIONS :

. It often manifests itself previously as chronic lacrimation. It may be congenital (3), in which case the obstruction of the nasolacrimal duct is congenital in origin, or it may be acquired, in which case the obstruction is secondary to chronic conjunctivolacrimal or post-traumatic infections causing a narrowing of the lacrimal ducts, leaving a narrowing at the entrance to the nasolacrimal duct.

Dacryocystitis is often diagnosed clinically. Acute dacryocystitis results in an abscess of the lacrimal sac, with pain and oedema of the internal palpebral angle, progressing to fistulisation. Chronic dacryocystitis, on the other hand, results in lacrimation that becomes purulent in the event of superinfection.

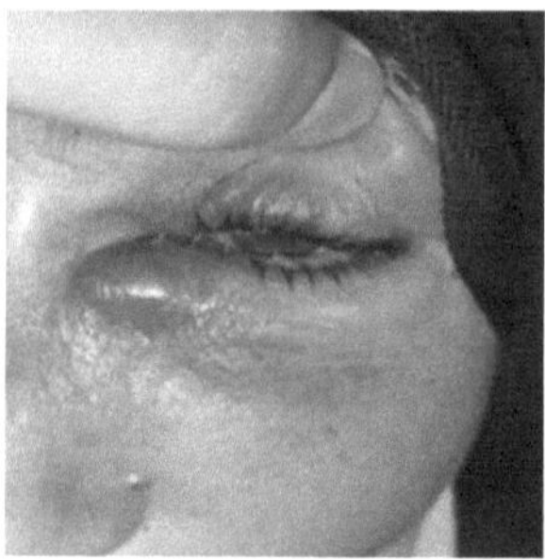

Figure 1: Acute dacryocystitis in a patient being treated for chronic rhino-conjunctivitis (Iconography by Pr F Mazari).

Probing of the lacrimal ducts reveals an obstruction, bringing back a few flakes of pus, suggesting the diagnosis. The most serious complication is corneal ulceration. In severe cases, orbital cellulitis and septicaemia may also occur.

The germs most frequently implicated were gram-positive germs (69%), followed by gram-negative germs (20%) and anaerobes (13%). Inflammation may be localised to the sac or accompanied by pericystitis, which may progress to chronicity; there is often preseptal cellulitis, but much more rarely orbital cellulitis with palpebral oedema, chemosis or ptosis. Orbital complications of dacryocystitis are rare due to anatomical barriers. The spontaneous evolution of the abscess may lead to resolution, often through fistulisation, or to resorption under appropriate antibiotic treatment.

TREATMENT :

. Medical treatment:

Broad-spectrum antibiotic therapy is administered systemically, in combination with local topical antibiotics, depending on the results of the antibiotic susceptibility test after secretions have been collected from the cul-de-sac or any skin fistula. The treatment that best covers the spectrum of germs usually responsible is a combination of a fluoroquinolone and a beta-lactam antibiotic or a third-generation cephalosporin and metronidazole. Non-steroidal anti-inflammatory drugs and analgesics should also be added. A dacryocystorhinostomy should be performed once the infection has been treated with antibiotics.

Surgical treatment :

The aim of surgical dacryocystorhinostomy is to bypass an obstacle in the lacrimonasal duct and allow tears to pass directly from the lacrimal sac into the nasal cavities. The two methods used are the external route and the endonasal route, which is mainly practised by ENT doctors.

REFERENCES

1. Adenis JP, Robert PY, Boncoeur-Martel MP. Anatomy of the lacrimal glands and ducts. Encycl Méd Chir Ophtalmologie, 1996;21-006-A25, 9p.
2. Ducasse A, Adenis J.P, Fayet B, George J.L, RubanJ.M. Les voies lacrymales. Paris, Masson, 2006, 640p.
3. Guez A, Dureau P. Larmoiement du nourrisson: conduite à tenir et thérapeutique. Arch Pédiatrie. 2009 May;16(5):496-9.
3. Piaton J.M, Keller P, Escals P. Pathology of the excretory lacrimal ducts (vertical portion). Diagnosis and treatment. EMC Ophthalmology 2006; 21- 175-A-30.
4. Baggio E, Ruban JM. Lacrimation with permeable tear ducts. Images en Ophtalmologie, Vol V (4) October-November-December 2011.

CELLULITIS ORBITAL

Introduction :

Orbital and periorbital cellulitis is one of the most common diagnostic and therapeutic emergencies in ophthalmology. A distinction is made between periorbital or pre septal cellulitis, located in front of the orbital septum, which is more common but less severe, and orbital or retro septal cellulitis, which is rare but has a poor prognosis. The seriousness of orbital cellulitis depends on its local, locoregional and general complications, with a compromised vital prognosis. The vital prognosis of these orbital cellulites is closely linked to the meninigo-encephalic complications. [The mortality rate varies from 5% to 25% in cases of associated intracranial complications [1,2]. Early diagnosis and immediate treatment are essential. Pathophysiology The onset of orbital cellulitis implies the presence of an infectious source, usually locoregional, in particular severe sinusitis and conjunctival or cutaneous infectious sources Orbital infections can be extensive and serious. Subperiosteal fluid collections, sometimes large, may form; these are known as subperiosteal abscesses. The Chandler Topographical and Clinical Classification summarises these different presentations.

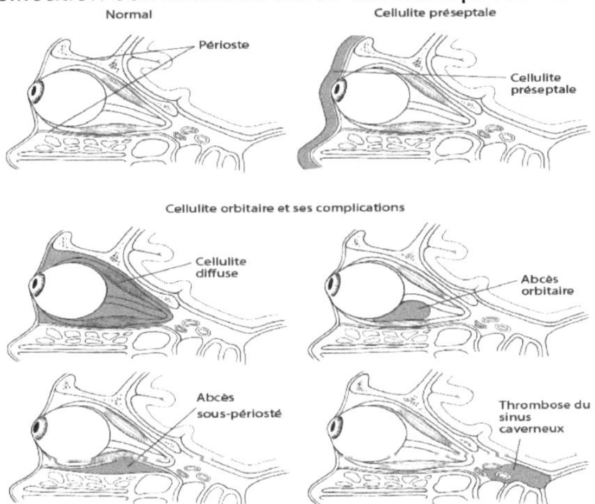

Figure 1: Pre-septal and orbital cellulitis: (Iconography reviewed in the literature).

Classification de **Chandler**: 5 stades par ordre de gravité croissante:

  • **Stade I**: cellulite préseptale: œdème inflammatoire de la paupière
  • **Stade II**: Cellulite orbitaire: oedème diffus orbitaire
  • **Stade III**: abcès sous périosté
  • **Stade IV**: abcès orbitaire
  • **Stade V**: thrombose du sinus caverneux

Table 1: Chandler's classification

Diagnosis :

Clinical :

Symptoms of preseptal cellulitis include pain, swelling, warmth and redness or discolouration (purplish in the case of H. influenzae infection) of the eyelid, and sometimes fever. Patients may not be able to open their eyes because the eyelid is swollen. The swelling and discomfort can make it difficult to examine the eye, but when it can be done, the examination shows that visual acuity is unaffected, ocular motility is intact and the globe is not pushed forward (exophthalmos).Clinical symptoms of orbital cellulitis include oedema and redness of the eyelid and adjacent soft tissues, conjunctival hyperaemia and chemosis, decreased and painful ocular motor activity, decreased visual acuity and exophthalmos caused by orbital swelling. Signs of primary infection are also often present (e.g. haemorrhage and nasal discharge with sinusitis, periodontal pain and enlargement associated with abscess). Fever is usually present. Headache and lethargy should raise suspicion of associated meningitis. Some or all of these symptoms may not be present in the early stages of infectionSubperiosteal abscesses, if large enough, can contribute to the symptoms of orbital cellulitis by causing swelling and redness of the eyelid, impaired ocular motor function, exophthalmos and reduced visual acuity. The diagnosis of preseptal cellulitis and orbital cellulitis is primarily clinical. The differential diagnosis to be considered includes trauma, insect bites without cellulitis, an intraorbital foreign body, an allergic reaction, tumours or an inflammatory orbital pseudotumour.Swelling of the eyelid may require the use of blepharostats to examine the globe, and early signs of complicated infection may be subtle. An ophthalmologist should be consulted if orbital cellulitis is suspected.The type of cellulitis, periorbital or orbital, can often be differentiated clinically. Periorbital cellulitis is likely if the ocular examination is normal, apart from palpebral swelling. The presence of a local infection on the skin makes periorbital cellulitis even more likely.If the signs are misleading, if examination is difficult (as in young children), or if there is a nasal discharge (suggesting sinusitis), a CT or MRI scan should be performed to rule out cellulitis, tumours and orbital pseudotumours. MRI is more appropriate than CT if thrombosis of the cavernous sinus is suspected.The direction of exophthalmos can be a clue to the site of infection; for example, extension from the frontal sinus pushes the globe down and out, and extension from the ethmoidal sinus pushes the globe laterally out.Blood cultures are often taken (ideally before starting antibiotics) in cases of orbital cellulitis, but less than 1/3 of them are positive. A lumbar puncture is performed if meningitis is suspected. Cultures of sinus fluid are taken if sinusitis is suspected as the starting point. Other laboratory tests are not particularly useful. The classic picture is that of a patient in a febrile state evolving in a context of altered general condition associated with significant inflammatory palpebral oedema.The Chandler classification (Table I) **is** used to classify the stages of cellulitis based on clinical examination.

Causes
Preseptal cellulitis is usually caused by the contiguous extension of infections due to local wounds of the face or eyelid or secondary to insect bites, animal bites, chalazion or sinusitis. Orbital cellulitis is most commonly caused by an extension of an infection of the adjacent sinuses, particularly the ethmoid sinus. Less commonly, orbital cellulitis is caused by direct infection accompanying local trauma (e.g. insect bite, animal bite, penetrating eyelid wounds) or by contiguous extension of infection from the face or teeth or spread by the haematogenous route. The pathogens vary according to the aetiology and age of the patient. Streptococcus pneumoniae is the most common pathogen associated with sinus infection, while Staphylococcus aureus and Streptococcus pyogenes predominate when the infection arises from local trauma.

Haemophilus influenzae type b, which used to be a frequent cause, is now less so due to widespread vaccination. Fungi are rare pathogens, responsible for orbital cellulitis in diabetics or immunocompromised patients. Infection in children aged < 9 years is generally due to a single aerobic microorganism; later on, particularly in patients aged > 15 years, the infection is usually mixed polymicrobial, aerobic and anaerobic (Bacteroides, Peptostreptococcus).

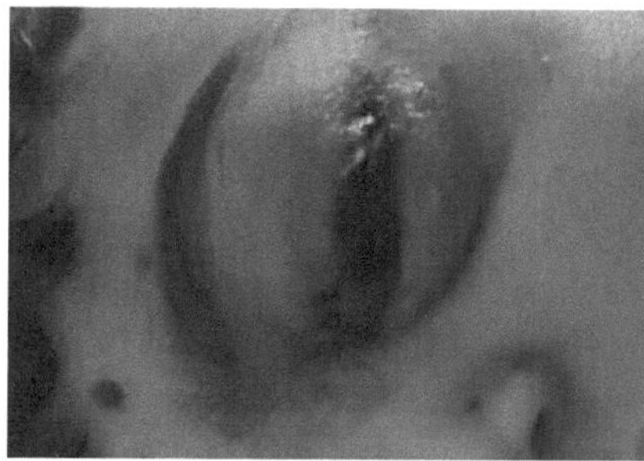

Figure 2- Orbital cellulitis in a 7-year-old child, following superinfection of a Varicella vesicle in the conjunctiva. (Iconography: Pr F Mazari).

Treatment :

1- Antibiotics :

•Pre-septal cellulitis :
In patients with preseptal cellulitis, initial treatment should be directed against the germs causing the sinusitis (S. pneumoniae, non-typeable H. influenzae, S. aureus, Moraxella catarrhalis); however, in areas where methicillin-resistant S. aureus is prevalent, the appropriate antibiotics should be added. appropriate antibiotics (p. eg, clindamycin, trimethoprim/sulfamethoxazole or doxycycline for oral treatment and vancomycin for inpatients). In the case of unclean wounds, a gram-negative infection should be suspected.

Outpatient treatment remains an option if orbital cellulitis has been definitively ruled out; children should show no signs of systemic infection and should be under the supervision of their parents or carers. Patients should be closely monitored by an ophthalmologist. Outpatient treatment options include amoxicillin/clavulanic acid 30mg/kg orally every 8 hours (in children <12 years) or 500mg orally every 8-12 hours or 875mg orally twice daily (in adults) for 10 days. (The dose may need to be increased if penicillin-resistant S. pneumoniae is suspected). In hospitalised patients, ampicillin/sulbactam 50 mg/kg IV every 6 hours (in children) or 1.5 to 3 g (in adults) IV every 6 hours (maximum 8 g ampicillin/day) for 7 days is an option. If S. aureus is resistant to methicillin, antibiotics should be adapted accordingly.

•Orbital cellulitis :

Patients with orbital cellulitis should be admitted to hospital and treated with meningitis dose antibiotics (see table Usual IV antibiotic doses for acute bacterial meningitis). A 2nd or 3rd generation cephalosporin, such as cefotaxime 50 mg/kg IV every 6 hours (in children < 12 years) or 1-2 g IV every 6 hours (in adults) for 14 days, is an option for sinusitis; imipenem, ceftriaxone and piperacillin/tazobactam are other alternatives. If the cellulitis is due to trauma or a foreign body, treatment must be effective against Gram-positive pathogens, including methicillin-resistant S. aureus in a prevalence area, (vancomycin 1 g IV every 12 hours) and Gram-negative pathogens (e.g. ertapenem 1 g IV once/day) and must be continued for 7 to 10 days or until clinical improvement (1). If anaerobic pathogens are suspected (as may be the case in dental infections), metronidazole is generally used.Surgery to decompress the orbit, drain an abscess, open an infected sinus or a combination of these procedures is indicated in any of the following circumstances:

- Vision is compromised.
- Suppuration or a foreign body is suspected.
- Imaging shows an orbital abscess or a large subperiosteal abscess, particularly along the orbital roof.
- The infection does not improve with antibiotics.

REFERENCES

1. Kahloun r, abroug n, abdessalem bn, ksiaa i, jelliti b, zaouali s et al. les infections orbitaires : à propos de 28 cas. la tunisie médicale 2015; 93(11): 673-7.

2. Belghmaidi s, belhoucha b, hajji i, hssaine k, rochdi y, nouri h et al. les cellulites orbitaires : étude prospective à propos de 75 cas. pan african medical journal 2015: 22: 340 doi:10.11604/pamj.2015.22.340.7279.

3. Bae c, bourget d. periorbital cellulitis. [updated 2020 jan 21] in: statpearls [internet]. treasure island (fl): statpearls publishing; 2020 jan-. available from: https://www.ncbi.nlm.nih.gov/books/ nbk 470408/.

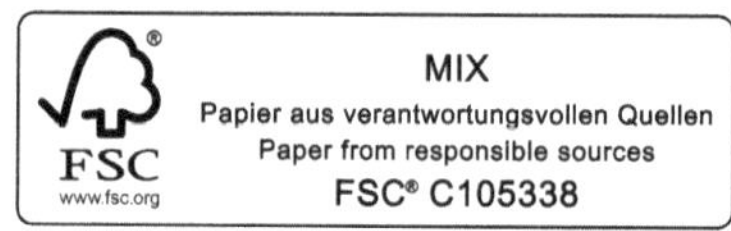

Printed by Books on Demand GmbH, Norderstedt / Germany